NO LONGER PROPERTY OF
ANYTHINK LIBRARIES/
RANGEVIEW LIBRARY DISTRICT

MANAGING CHRONIC PAIN IN AN AGE OF ADDICTION

MANAGING CHRONIC PAIN IN AN AGE OF ADDICTION

Akhtar Purvez, MD
Foreword by John Rowlingson, MD

ROWMAN & LITTLEFIELD
Lanham • Boulder • New York • London

Medicine is a science and an art. A clinician-patient relationship is fundamental to the arrangement that is necessary to offering and receiving medical care. Patients are advised to consult a qualified clinician for any medical needs and advice. This book is meant to be an authoritative account of issues related to chronic pain and addiction. The information provided should not be construed as medical advice and no such relationship is or should be implied. The author and publisher do not take any responsibility for any consequences resulting from utilization of any information presented in this book.

Published by Rowman & Littlefield
An imprint of The Rowman & Littlefield Publishing Group, Inc.
4501 Forbes Boulevard, Suite 200, Lanham, Maryland 20706
www.rowman.com

Unit A, Whitacre Mews, 26-34 Stannary Street, London SE11 4AB

Copyright © 2018 by The Rowman & Littlefield Publishing Group, Inc.

All rights reserved. No part of this book may be reproduced in any form or by any electronic or mechanical means, including information storage and retrieval systems, without written permission from the publisher, except by a reviewer who may quote passages in a review.

British Library Cataloguing in Publication Information Available

Library of Congress Cataloging-in-Publication Data

Names: Purvez, Akhtar, author.
Title: Managing chronic pain in an age of addiction / Akhtar Purvez.
Description: Lanham : Rowman & Littlefield, [2018] | Includes bibliographical references and index.
Identifiers: LCCN 2018012528 (print) | LCCN 2018012053 (ebook) | ISBN 9781538109236 (cloth : alk. paper) | ISBN 9781538109243 (Electronic)
Subjects: | MESH: Pain Management—methods | Chronic Pain—drug therapy | Chronic Pain—complications | Analgesics, Opioid—adverse effects | Opioid-Related Disorders—prevention & control | Behavior, Addictive—prevention & control
Classification: LCC RB127 (ebook) | LCC RB127 (print) | NLM WL 704.6 | DDC 616/.0472—dc23
LC record available at https://lccn.loc.gov/2018012528

∞ ™ The paper used in this publication meets the minimum requirements of American National Standard for Information Sciences Permanence of Paper for Printed Library Materials, ANSI/NISO Z39.48-1992.

Printed in the United States of America

To my patients and their families for their perseverance, patience and courage.

CONTENTS

FOREWORD

All of us have experienced acute pain from an injury or surgery. The pain provoked a visit to a doctor or a hospital, the diagnosis was made, treatment was provided, and the pain disappeared after a short time. That is hardly the course for patients with chronic pain. Their pain *lingers*, and it becomes harder to deal with as time passes. Treatments that ease acute pain don't always work for chronic pain, creating friction between the patient and the prescribing doctor, who may not be trained to manage chronic pain. What's worse is that the *enduring* nature of chronic pain results in changes in the patient's attitude about ever getting healthy again, dramatic behaviors that are fueled by the patient's frustration at the persistence of pain in spite of treatment, and major lifestyle disruptions, such as limiting the patient's ability to go to work. While these events play on the patients and the loved ones supporting them, anxiety, depression, and other psychological effects become more prevalent and interfere with their day-to-day existence. As if these consequences aren't enough trouble, chronic pain actually leads to changes in the function of the patient's nervous system, almost assuring that the pain will persist.

One of the key elements of chronic pain management is the evaluation of the patient to establish what's actually causing the pain. This process must investigate all dimensions of the patient's being, including the physical, emotional, social, economic, and spiritual realms. The patient must be fully open with the physician about the history of the pain.

The physical examination documents the muscle, joint, and nerve changes related to the original injury, previous surgery, or the limitations induced by the ongoing pain. Laboratory test results can be very disappointing since the studies don't prove the intensity or the presence of pain, nor necessarily support the patient's perceived or actual disability. Unfortunately, we do not have a convenient numerical guide, like high blood pressure values or blood sugar levels in diabetes, to measure the impact of chronic pain on the patient's life. The use of simple word or number scales to assess chronic pain does not delve far enough into how much the chronic pain disrupts the patient's life to provide an adequate picture of the harm.

The doctor must detect how the pain is interfering with the patient's ability to function, handle his or her emotions on a daily basis, stay clearheaded in spite of pain medications, and enjoy meaningful activities with family, friends, and coworkers. Just taking the chronic pain away does not solve all of the pain-related issues. Thus, the patient needs *both* a thorough evaluation *and* a dynamic pain management plan that targets all of the identified contributors to the pain *and* prepares the patients to be improved.

Chronic pain is rarely cured, so the patient must adopt the concept of managing it as a disease, like diabetes or asthma. The overall goal of pain treatment is to decrease the intensity and the frequency of the pain so that the patient's quality of life and ability to function can be enriched. The good news is that most patients will see these benefits from the *treatment program*—the coordinated use of a number of different modalities to minimize the likelihood of treatment side effects but that, when used together, create a sustained decrease in pain. The use of medications alone will not be successful. They have many side effects including dependence and addiction. Patients enjoy freedom from pill taking when they embrace physical therapy, yoga, meditation, and other treatments described in this book that address more of the disease elements of their chronic pain.

This book is a breath of fresh air among the innumerable textbooks dealing with pain management. The text is written in the style of a direct, honest conversation with the patient, resulting in the patient's *understanding* of the chronic pain. It anticipates the patient's questions and provides the answers in a straightforward dialogue. It communicates in the language of the average patient to explain why the pain persists and doesn't merely go away. This book is wide ranging in its coverage of essential topics that the author genuinely wants the patient to comprehend. It broadcasts the message that while all pain may not disappear, modern-day treatment helps the patient cope with leftover pain.

This book acknowledges that chronic pain is not only the patient's problem. The book will beckon those who have lost their social network and have replaced their independence with reliance on others. It will have a life-changing impact on patients *and* their caregivers, so that the evils of chronic pain have a lesser hold on their lives. The book's content will impart valuable knowledge so that patients *and* their doctors will not make decisions about pain management in the unhealthy mind-set of desperation. The book highlights that there is so much more to be done for pain management than just providing medications and that the patient *can* regain control of the pain.

Dr. Purvez is a thoughtful, steadfast, qualified pain management physician, teacher, researcher, and pain management advocate. His life is guided by a spiritual upbringing that fosters his patience, humility, and compassion. He has respect for all people so that biases do not determine which patients he will treat nor the treatment options he will offer. He favors patient evaluations that are insightful and treatment plans that are rational, ethically sound, and relevant to *the* issues identified. His generosity is shown in the creation of this book because it shares his successful personal approach to chronic pain management with patients *and* caregivers across the healthcare spectrum. Indeed, the book will be valuable to those with pain management experience who are looking for a more effective communication rhetoric *and* those not trained in chronic pain management but who are eager to serve these patients.

Dr. Purvez's ambition is to enhance everyone's understanding of chronic pain—a most complicated, worldwide health issue. He has created a book that is comprehensive in its scope yet gentle in its prose. Thanks to Dr. Purvez for his incredible effort to raise pain control beyond merely pill bottles and needles. This readable book will be of help to countless patients and their families because they will grasp more of what makes chronic pain so difficult, *and* it will be of help to their doctors, who will become aware of the numerous therapies to reduce chronic pain.

John C. Rowlingson, MD
Cosmo A. DiFazio, Professor of Anesthesiology
Department of Anesthesiology
University of Virginia School of Medicine

ACKNOWLEDGMENTS

This book was written over a decade, during which my thought process in general, and the concept of pain management in particular, evolved fundamentally. I have many people to thank for their contribution.

My own family has always been there for me on every step of my career and my life. My wife is a source of constant inspiration, unconditional love, and support. A physician, she put her own career on hold during my tough training years in America. My children offer additional affection and warmth at home, which negates the stress outside of it. My parents and my brother give constant love and encouragement. My father, who is a poet, an author, and an intellectual, has been and continues to be a role model. Without all this, my journey would have been much more challenging, if not entirely impossible.

I owe great credit to Dr. John Rowlingson, a thought leader, my mentor, friend, and guide, who taught me not just the fundamentals of pain management but also much of the art of patient care. He recommended me for my first job, kept me inspired, and was kind enough to write the foreword for this book. I deeply appreciate his guidance at every point.

Robert Darrell Laurant is a man with qualities that only a few are born with—humility, clear and concise thinking, and an amazingly creative mind. For years, the first thing I did every morning was to enjoy his daily column in the local newspaper. It was an honor to have him as a researcher and editor of this book. I cannot thank him enough for the hard work he put forth to bring this project to fruition.

I am grateful to numerous nursing, imaging, and ancillary colleagues with whom I have had the pleasure to work over the years and who helped me appreciate the value of compassion and the team approach, which is essential to optimizing patient care. My special thanks go to my physician colleagues, past and at my present place of work, who have helped me grow personally and professionally.

Ana Mir offered constructive criticism and advice from a journalistic viewpoint that helped guide the course of this book. Sama Mir, Guleer Shahab, Nicole Apicella, Najeeha Khan, and Ameera Farooqi were essential to the editing and research process that made this project what it turned out to be.

This book would not have been possible without the express help, advice, and support of Suzanne I. Staszak-Silva, executive editor at Rowman & Littlefield. She is a brilliant, no-nonsense, can-do publisher who was instrumental in guiding a novice writer to a published one.

INTRODUCTION: A LONG WAY FROM KASHMIR

We gashed mountains' chests to satiate our tulips—
and adorned our land with pearls of morning dew.
We savored life and kept the pledge of love.
 —From the poem "Wize Wize" by Kashmiri poet, Muzaffar Aazim

I grew up in a place that humbles people.

Human arrogance quickly evaporates at the sight of the Himalayas, mountains grand enough to bridge heaven and earth. Whether one is Hindu, Muslim, Christian, or Buddhist, it's easy to imagine your particular deity seated on a rocky throne somewhere above the clouds.

Small wonder that the lands known collectively as the Roof of the World—Nepal, Tibet, parts of Pakistan, India, and China, as well as my native Kashmir—are also known for their monks, gurus, fakirs, and shrines. We are Jacks living in the shadow of the beanstalk; awed worshippers at a massive, snow-capped altar.

Although these images tend to make Kashmir seem cold and stark, nothing could be further from the truth. There, nature has thoughtfully laid out a series of fertile, welcoming valleys that gradually ascend the foothills of the great mountains in verdant bands. These valleys enfold diverse, warm, and welcoming groups of people, places where the inhabitants have learned to live side by side in peace. In the tumultuous years surrounding independence from the British, when the whole subcontinent was engulfed in darkness, hatred, and sectorial violence, Mahatma Gandhi, the epitome of ahimsa, or nonviolence, saw a "ray of hope in Kashmir."[1] There is something about a valley, especially one walled in by high peaks. The people there are like different ingredients poured into a vessel and allowed to marinate. In the Kashmir of my youth, where modern-day amenities were more the exception than the rule, that enforced togetherness was emphasized even more.

True, things have changed tremendously since that semi-idyllic childhood. There have been outward stresses to the Kashmiri brand of tranquility (mostly territorial squabbles between the larger Indian nation and surrounding countries), interior tension between different groups, and turbulence caused by Kashmiris seeking more freedom from their Indian-based government.

For the Muslims, followers of what is the majority religion in Kashmir, nothing in their religious teaching advocated violence or dismissed any other religions as inferior. There were no impassioned calls to conversion by force, no brutality toward women. There was peace and contentment.

The faith that fed me was primarily about how to live a life of service and kindness toward everyone. One that respects the rights and points of view of others. It also mixed reason and moderation in with that spirituality, making it an ideal path for a physician to tread.

Perhaps individual religions become more militant when they are the only alternative, when any other way of life or pattern of thought is unimaginable. Although there are more Muslims than anything else in Kashmir, the population must also associate, interact, and conduct business with members of a dozen other denominations and sects. Our ancient river of history is fed by many streams of culture, from Genghis Khan to the British colonialists.

It is a magical place, and the longer I live in other places, the stronger that magic becomes.

For a few years, I attended a missionary school founded by British Christians and then a so-called Anglo-Vedic school that promoted a perfect blend of modern Western and classic Eastern culture. Both schools emphasized morality but no particular religious teaching.

More recently, Kashmir has seen long periods of violence, death, and destruction. The name "Kashmir" now brings forth images of burning buildings, shaken innocent and hopeless children, and grim-faced infantrymen. In the public mind, this is the obscure corner of the planet that almost triggered the world's first war between two nuclear powers, India and Pakistan. A place to stay far, far away from.

It's true that the area's key geographic position has made it a bone of contention, to be claimed by three contending countries—India, Pakistan, and China—all of whom control parts of the state. For a long time, their pride has prevented them from coming to a solution. When I think of my homeland, however, I prefer to remember that Kashmir was the setting for the 1930s novel *Lost Horizons*, which gave the world the mythical paradise known as Shangri-la.

For what it's worth, Kashmir is also known for birthing the cashmere sweater and inspiring a hit song by the iconic rock group Led Zeppelin. And I suppose it is a compliment of sorts that so many countries want to claim it for their own. Everyone wants the key to Shangri-la.

The reality of Kashmir sits somewhere between chaos and paradise. When I moved to the United States as a young man, the contrast between cultures made me realize the poverty that once surrounded me. But it was a poverty of possessions, not of spirit.

Of course, you know from this book's title that it is not about Kashmir. It is a book about pain. I mention my origins only because they have much to do with my current attitudes as a human being and as a physician. I now work and live in Virginia, but the compassion and patience critical for my specialty had already been bestowed upon me back in that high mountain valley.

Along with the aforementioned humility, doctors are respected in Kashmir and most undoubtedly bask in that respect. With their station in life, however, comes an unspoken prohibition against any form of bragging or self-promotion.

When I was looking for my first medical residency training position in the United States, I was asked by one interviewer: "So, why should we hire you for this position?" I was dumbfounded. I had thought my résumé spoke for itself, and I wasn't prepared to list all my accomplishments out loud. It seemed like boasting.

At the time, the first thing on my résumé was my name, age, father's name, and address. My awards, honors, and accomplishments were far down at the bottom. Soon I realized I needed to present and highlight the latter and flip-flop that original order completely.

I'm not saying one way is better than another, just that it's different in America.

My goal with this book is to communicate in some meaningful way with the average reader, whether that person is suffering from chronic pain or is close to someone else residing in that unpleasant space. For while there is no lack of information about pain in libraries and on the Internet, much of it is either highly technical and designed for physicians or too vague for the general public.

Chances are a person in pain isn't all that interested in how the nociceptors and inhibitory cells collaborate (or don't collaborate) with the cerebral cortex. That person wants to know why he or she hurts, but only on a practical level. The most important question to be answered is: "How can I fix this?" If the response is "You can't," the next question is: "Then how can I learn to live with this to get the most out of my life?"

We, as doctors, sometimes try to dance around the reality of pain, choosing what we think are more palatable euphemisms.

"You might feel some discomfort," we say, or, "There might be a little pressure."

I believe in honesty and in getting to know my patients as individuals I can look in the face. In return, I think it's only fair that they, and the readers of this book, learn a little about me.

My family was not wealthy in terms of money but had significant land holdings in the lower (seven thousand feet) Kashmir Valley. Many people rented land from us and used it to grow their own crops. We called them *tillers*. Later, I learned that the American term was *share-croppers*. Unlike in the United States, however, we considered them partners rather than employees, and we split the value of the crops they raised roughly fifty-fifty.

Government land reform in the 1950s and 1960s took most of those holdings away from my grandfather, the family patriarch, but we still managed to make a living. Then, as now, agriculture is the main source of income in the Kashmir valleys, and we retained enough land to grow food for our own subsistence. All the family members participated in the growing and harvesting, and the only things our land didn't provide for us were salt, kerosene for lighting, and soap. Those we bought at a small local store.

Health care, as one might expect, was problematic. As a child in the late 1960s, I remember that the nearest doctor was ten miles from our house. Anyone hoping to summon him would ride a horse to the doctor's house, then walk while the physician rode back to his "horse call."

That seems quaint today, even for Kashmir, but the province is still lagging behind in advanced and tertiary care facilities. Those who can afford it travel to places like Delhi, the capital of India, for medical care. Engulfed in political turmoil, the state does not get all the support it needs from the federal government.

Given my sympathy for the country of my birth and its underserved inhabitants, I am sometimes asked why I don't return to Kashmir to practice medicine. Part of me might be fulfilled by that, but the reality is that Kashmir still does not have the resources and setup necessary to practice my specialty efficiently there. I'm not sure how much good I could do.

Yet the seeds to my eventual life's work were sown there as a child, when I would see people in pain, suffering only because there was no medical help available. I was like young Buddha, deeply distressed by the suffering and intent on doing something about it when I grew up. The nearest clinical health facility was twenty-five miles away, the closest full-service hospital more than fifty. Local herbal and natural remedies sometimes worked (and I'm not one to debunk them) but often did not.

Meanwhile, growing up amid the human diversity of Kashmir taught me that all people who feel pain are the same, whether they are suffering in a poverty-stricken corner of Asia or an affluent American suburb. Pain is nothing if not democratic, unimpressed by bank account or social standing.

Becoming a doctor was always a dream of mine, and my father provided an excellent example of chasing dreams. When the loss of land through government reform required that some of our family members find "outside" jobs, he became the director of sericulture in Kashmir. He is an intellectual, and his dream and focus are art, literature, and poetry. He made a decision to follow that dream and took an early retirement from his high-status job to do just that, to the amazement of his coworkers and friends. He went on to write many books and translate landmark pieces of literature like Leo Tolstoy's *War and Peace* and Emily Brontë's *Wuthering Heights* into Kashmiri. My brother was drawn to immigration law, and my parents encouraged him to seek further schooling in America.

Similarly, I saw medicine as a logical destination where I would be able to offer my best to those who needed it most.

Our parents instilled in us the virtues of honesty, hard work, service, and respect for our fellow human being—the priceless gifts that have always guided our lives through thick and thin.

As it turned out, the first year I spent as a surgical resident in New York City almost changed my mind. The brutal and grueling schedule required of residents at that time seemed designed to weed out those of weaker will, and it often worked. I remember asking about another promising young man from Kashmir who had chosen the same path before me and being told, "He's already gone. He only lasted about two months."

Which is not surprising, given the up to twenty-hour shifts we had to endure. Most days, I remember getting to bed after midnight and then arising at 4:00 a.m. to make hospital rounds. I remember having to decide between eating and sleeping, reasoning that the half hour it would take to prepare dinner might be better spent on rest. It is here that the patience and perseverance I developed in my formative years paid off. It was baptism by fire.

In recent years, hospital administrators finally came to the realization that being attended by sleep-deprived, hollow-eyed residents might not be best for the patients, and the schedule was moderated. By then, however, it was only a bad memory for me.

My next three years were spent in Boston, studying anesthesiology and learning much of what I now know about pain and how to confront it.

The anesthesiologist's job is a study in balance. If the patient on the operating table is not sufficiently sedated, he or she might still feel pain during the procedure. Conversely, oversedating a patient can, in rare cases, be fatal.

True, we have considerable control about how much of a drug is administered. Still, tragic accidents happen, and no one wants to have to tell a grieving family, "The operation was a success, but the patient died."

Most unnerving for me were the few times when the person on the operating table appeared to be possibly aware, judging from the vital signs, even though the patient's muscles were paralyzed by the anesthesia and he or she was unable to respond. That was quickly fixed by an adjustment in anesthetic level, but even a brief glimpse into what could have possibly been sheer torture was haunting.

I had many options to continue my clinical education in pain medicine after anesthesiology school, including at Georgetown, Harvard, and Johns Hopkins. In the end, I chose the University of Virginia because of John Rowlingson. He is an authority on pain medicine and widely known for his expertise, skill, and compassion. He is the author of significant scientific papers and book chapters and a frequent speaker at national medical seminars, conventions, and workshops.

Rowlingson might be best known for working on a Virginia governor's board and steering a law allowing physicians to prescribe opioid medications for more than just cancer pain. That commonsense measure has since been adopted by all forty-nine other states.

I now practice in Charlottesville, Virginia. It is a beautiful town nestled in mountains and one that is home to Thomas Jefferson's University of Virginia, my alma mater. As a Virginian, I am proud that this fertile state produced eight of the forty-five U.S. presidents.

However, my first job was in Lynchburg, Virginia. I dictated most of this book on my one-and-a-half-hour drive to and from work. Looking back, this was a blessing in disguise. In what other setup would I have the luxury of three hours each day to think and write?

It was also Rowlingson who told me shortly before my graduation from the University of Virginia Medical School that a major hospital group in the city of Lynchburg, seventy miles to the south of Charlottesville, was looking for a pain specialist.

In time, I learned that Lynchburg has a remarkable medical history. Established by Quakers in the late 1700s, it became a major treatment center for battlefield casualties and victims of disease during the American Civil War, when more than a dozen of its tobacco factories were converted into hospitals. One of those Quaker descendants, Dr. John Jay Terrell, worked with smallpox patients at a small facility that became known as the "Pest House" and contributed significantly to our knowledge of how best to treat infectious diseases.

Even so, the idea of commuting over an hour and a half in each direction was daunting. Rowlingson urged me to try it, and I did. With time, I began to find the drive more productive and restorative than grueling, passing as it does through pastoral landscapes framed by the Blue Ridge Mountains.

Mountains almost as beautiful as those in Kashmir.

I

MEDICATIONS THAT RELIEVE PAIN— AND KILL

WHAT DO PHYSICIANS RECOMMEND FIRST?

Keeping track of the multitude of drugs that purport to ease chronic pain has become almost a full-time job for chronic pain specialists.

Medical research is in a constant state of hyperactivity, its practitioners always hoping to convert weeks and months of exhaustive tests into a new approach, a new drug, or even word of a new disease. Not a month goes by without some groundbreaking revelation being brought forth at a press conference or in an article published by one of the leading medical journals.

What is the practicing physician to do with this constant barrage of new information and new products? As might be expected, there is always the push and pull between not wanting to miss a possible opportunity and a natural caution toward something new and relatively unproven.

For drugs are, after all, a commercial product. If one company develops a pill that seems effective for sufferers of fibromyalgia, other companies will see the financial possibilities and redouble their efforts to put out an even better fibromyalgia drug. Somewhere in all the competing television ads, medical common sense can get lost.

Even so, it would be a lot easier if all patients reacted to medication in the same way. Then, it would simply be a matter of figuring out what seems to be the best shingles drug out of all the possible choices and prescribing it—a time-consuming process, perhaps, but still a matter of always plugging A into B.

Alas, we human beings are not assembly line products. What works for one patient may do nothing for another. A tolerable dose for one person could lead to overdose in another.

Nevertheless, some people tend to want a magic bullet. They ask: "Isn't there something you can give me for this?"

Usually, there is. But I have also learned over the years that medication is but one of the multiple options available to improve the life of those in chronic pain. Often with these patients it is more beneficial to shift the focus of treatment to approaches such as a course of physical therapy followed by regular physical exercise and specifically targeted procedures and nerve blocks.

A vigorously enforced daily exercise schedule is what improves their range of motion, builds their core, eases the reflex muscle spasm, and eases their pain. These, in combination, improve their quality of life. And that is what most patients need to hear, but some don't want to.

Medications may be useful to ward off severe pain in the short term, to stabilize a patient so that he or she can begin physical therapy, or to lower pain to a tolerable level. Rarely do medications make chronic pain go away for even a short time, and even more rarely do they make it stop.

It would be impossible—and unwise—for me to ignore medications altogether, yet they should be seen as a means to an end, not the end itself. The target must be the root cause of the pain if possible, whether the weapon is an anti-inflammatory drug, a muscle relaxant, or something for nerve pain like an antidepressant or an antiseizure medication. In many instances, this medication needs to instituted in combination with an interventional procedure such as nerve blocks, ablation, or pain-modulating implants.

Simple and commonly available medications such as acetaminophen can be used without a prescription. Other over-the-counter medications such as naproxen and ibuprofen are frequently recommended and may be sufficiently effective for minor to moderate pain.

Still, even these simple drugs can lead to serious side effects, including organ damage or death. Take, for example, acetaminophen. This drug has been available over the counter for many decades now and is commonly used for fever and pain. And while it is an effective medication, its downside can be a major concern.

A normal adult human body can metabolize a maximum of four grams, or an equivalent of eight extra-strength acetaminophen tablets, in twenty-four hours. Beyond that, this medication can lead to severe liver damage and death. The new guidelines limit the amount of this medication to not more than six extra-strength tablets in twenty-four hours, around three thousand milligrams. In addition, we need to realize that more than 50 percent of other cold and cough medications sold over the counter may also contain acetaminophen. It is the combination of these medications together in higher dosages that has resulted in most cases of acetaminophen liver damage and death.

"Data compiled by the U.S. Food and Drug Administration has linked as many as 980 deaths in a year to drugs containing acetaminophen. In addition, FDA reports of death associated with acetaminophen have been increasing faster than those for aspirin, ibuprofen and many other common over-the-counter pain medicines."[1]

Meanwhile, naproxen and ibuprofen are in a class of powerful drugs known as nonsteroidal anti-inflammatory medications. They can also reduce fever and pain and may be beneficial for injuries or for the relief of inflammatory processes like degenerative disc disease and osteoarthritis. Side effects, however, can include stomach upset, ulcers, and kidney damage, which could prove fatal. "Conservative calculations estimate that approximately 107,000 patients are hospitalized annually for nonsteroidal anti-inflammatory drug (NSAID)–related gastrointestinal (GI) complications and at least 16,500 NSAID-related deaths occur each year among arthritis patients alone."[2]

The same also applies to pain-relief powders such as BC, which contains aspirin, salicylamide, and caffeine. These may be effective in keeping minor pain under control in recommended amounts but could also lead to the same unintended consequences as the anti-inflammatory drugs discussed above.

In 1986, the World Health Organization (WHO) came out with a three-step ladder for cancer pain:

If pain occurs, there should be prompt oral administration of drugs in the following order: nonopioids (aspirin and paracetamol); then, as necessary, mild opioids (codeine); then strong opioids such as morphine, until the patient is free of pain. To calm fears and anxiety, additional drugs—"adjuvants"—should be used.

To maintain freedom from pain, drugs should be given "by the clock," that is every 3–6 hours, rather than "on demand." This three-step approach of administering the right drug in the right dose at the right time is inexpensive and 80–90% effective. Surgical intervention on appropriate nerves may provide further pain relief if drugs are not wholly effective.[3]

The new fourth step was then recommended, which included some injections and nerve blocks.

Over time, there has been considerable debate and doubt about whether "the Ladder" is a safe approach for noncancer pain given the ongoing serious death and devastation from the opioid crisis. In addition, there is new research that suggests that many other nonopioid medications may be equally, if not more, effective for many cases of chronic pain.

A host of such new drugs are being developed. These include a class of anti-inflammatory drugs known as COX-2 inhibitors. These drugs specifically inhibit the enzyme COX-2, which causes inflammation. These did fall into disrepute because of serious cardiovascular risks such as stroke and heart attacks, which led to the withdrawal of two out of three such medications. However, the last of the three drugs, celecoxib, is currently available and approved by the U.S. Food and Drug Administration (FDA). We now know that other, older anti-inflammatory drugs can also have similar side effects and that due prudence is necessary when prescribing these or other medications that may appear to be harmless.

Opium has been used historically for pain relief and, by some, for its mind-altering effect. Opioids, on the other hand, are drugs that have opium-like effects but are mostly synthetic and are now used only for the relief of pain. We now have dozens of newer semisynthetic and synthetic drugs in this class, and new drugs are being created as we go.

Opioids are very strong pain-relieving medications—in expert hands, they are valuable instruments in treating both acute and chronic pain. Unfortunately, with this potency comes strong side effects that may result in fatal respiratory failure. In addition, this class of drugs are strongly addicting. Addiction often leaves its victims dysfunctional, not to mention prime candidates for a lethal overdose and death from this drug or from a combination of other drugs, substances, and alcohol. Over sixty-four thousand people died this way in the United States in 2016 alone, emphasizing the need for a major paradigm shift and new, stricter regulations.[4] Some overdoses are suicidal, of course, but most are accidental. We've all read about the celebrities and movie stars such as Marilyn Monroe, Michael Jackson, Heath Ledger, Judy Garland, and Phillip Seymour Hoffman whose lives were cut down in their prime. And then there are over sixty-four thousand people just from the year 2016 who have remained unnamed.

The effects of opioids can be illustrated on a bell curve, and on the downward swing of that curve lurks death.

The number and type of opioids that are available to a treating healthcare provider are large and expanding. The basic morphine is still prescribed, most effectively in solution as in the morphine pump, often hooked up at the bedside of postoperative patients. In addition, opioids can be used orally or topically. Other such medications include methadone, oxycodone, hydrocodone, hydromorphone, fentanyl, buprenorphine, oxymorphone, and tapentadol.

When patients are seen in chronic pain management centers, they are required to sign a contract focusing on guidelines for taking opioid medications. With this comes instructions on how to use—and not use—these medications, especially as to how they might react with other medications. This also includes consent to monitoring and drug screening, which is routinely, and randomly, performed.

By law, these patients' prescription history is checked regularly through a prescription drug-monitoring program, which is available in forty-nine states. Most states monitor DEA (U.S. Drug Enforcement Administration) Schedule II to IV, which include opioids, ketamine, anabolic steroids, anxiety, and sleep medications. Schedule I are substances that have no current medical use but high abuse potential and include LSD, marijuana, heroin, and ecstasy. Schedule V are drugs like Lyrica and Lomotil that have low abuse potential. Lyrica is a drug approved for the relief of pain associated with diabetes, fibromyalgia, postherpetic neuralgia (PHN), and spinal cord injury. Lomotil is a medication used for the management of diarrhea.

Many states, including Virginia, where I practice, now also monitor gabapentin. This is not an opioid or benzodiazepine but an antiseizure drug that has nerve-pain-relieving properties. It is indicated for epilepsy and postherpetic neuralgia but is now being used as a mood stabilizer and for other conditions like diabetic neuropathy, sciatica, and restless leg syndrome. In recent years, gabapentin has turned into a drug of abuse, possibly related to euphoria, relaxation, and a "high" that patients experience especially in combination with opioids.

Given that some patients may turn out to be irresponsible stewards of their medications, many opioid medications are now presented in an abuse-resistant form that prevents certain ingredients from being separated out. Some formulations are crush resistant or combined with a reversing agent. In some, niacin is added, which causes severe itching if the drug is abused.

A patient seated in a doctor's office can look at pain medications quite logically and leave with the best of intentions. The test comes later, when that person is alone and chronic pain is bearing down on them. When the pain is at its worst, an overdose might seem like a small risk to take on the road to relief but it can end in disaster.

Nothing destroys logic faster than pain.

As we will discuss in the next section of this chapter, the medications that heal can also kill.

OPIOID PAIN DRUGS: THE DARK SIDE

On the surface, there is nothing easier than writing a prescription—a couple of scribbles, a quick flip of the wrist to separate sheet from pad, an extended hand. And more recently, no more than just a few clicks of the mouse.

If the recipient is a chronic pain patient, however, this simple transaction can be a moment of profound anticipation. Chances are, many other medications have already failed, yet there is always the hope that this will be the one to restore a normal life.

For the physician, conversely, there is often a lurking sense of uneasiness. Perhaps gun shop owners—the responsible ones, anyway—have the same feeling when they hand over their merchandise.

Much can go right with today's drugs, but much can also go wrong. With first-time patients, I can only assume that they will follow my instructions and the instructions on the bottle and not take too much— or combine them with other drugs, alcohol, or other substances. If the medication is an opioid, I trust that it will be used for pain relief and not recreation or the search for forgetfulness.

Increasingly, these are too many ifs for the average physician, which is why many of the stronger medications for chronic pain are now most often prescribed by pain specialists. With the recent emphasis on the devastating opioid crisis in the nation and the availability of a wide range of evidence-based interventional approaches, fortunately the ranks of those physicians prescribing heavy doses of opioid medications are dwindling instead of increasing.

Most of the patients who come to see me are genuinely and honestly seeking the relief of their symptoms and to be able to again enjoy their daily activities and be productive members of society. However, I do see some with questionable intentions, to say the least.

A few years back, a patient traveled almost two hundred miles to see me for chronic pain. He said that his prescribing physician had lost his license to practice—a red flag. This patient had upper back and neck pain that radiated down his right arm. He had not had any physical therapy or nerve blocks and was not on any anti-inflammatory drugs or nerve pain medications that are commonly prescribed for this condition. Instead, he was on a very heavy and deadly regimen of opioid medications that included methadone, oxycodone, and hydromorphone. A thorough evaluation and assessment of documentation and imaging revealed a localized cervical spine disc issue that was pressing on a nerve. I suggested physical therapy and a trial of epidural steroid injections and explained to him that his next step might be a surgical correction. I also informed him that he had very good chances of recovery with surgery, with the possibility of complete relief of pain. I offered to facilitate this process for him. However, the patient refused and insisted that I write a prescription for the heavy opioid medications that he had been prescribed for many years. It was hard for me to believe that he was actually taking that amount of medication, which would have easily killed a large animal with a single dose. I strongly suspected diversion of medications, and following my Hippocratic Oath of "first do no harm," I refused to write the prescriptions he was asking for. Obviously, the patient was not happy with the plan I had offered, but I know I made the right decision.

Back in early 2001, when I was undergoing fellowship training in pain management at the University of Virginia, we were told that less than 1 percent of chronic pain patients on opioid medications get addicted and that this number was higher in the general population. This conclusion, which sounds genuinely off now, was mainly based on just one reference connected to a letter to the *New England Journal of Medicine* in 1980. Another report from 1986 concluded that for cancer, pain narcotics can be "safely and effectively prescribed to patients with relatively little risks of producing maladaptive behavior which define opioid abuse."[5]

Big pharmaceutical companies funded institutions like the American Pain Society, previously headed by Dr. Russell Portenoy, that reported on low addiction potential and recommended expanding narcotic prescribing.

In the year 2001, the Joint Commission on Accreditation of Healthcare Organizations (JCAHO) introduced pain as the fifth vital sign to prioritize its treatment. According to a report in the *New Yorker*,[6] Purdue Pharma, a major drug company, helped fund a "pain management program" through the Joint Commission that may have facilitated the drug company's access to hospitals to promote OxyContin. The *New Yorker* report also mentions a policy drafted by several people with ties to narcotics makers, including J. David Haddox of the Federation of State Medical Boards, that called on the state boards to punish doctors for inadequately treating pain. This apparent collaboration between Big Pharma and academics might have been the watershed moment that has resulted in the massive crisis that is related to the current opioid epidemic. Purdue Pharma pled guilty to criminal charges that they had misled the FDA, clinicians, and patients about the risks of OxyContin addiction and abuse by aggressively marketing the drug to providers and patients as a safe alternative to short-acting narcotics, as reported by the *New Yorker*.

So here we are, in 2017, faced with a massive addicted population and limited resources to manage pain. Leaving the blame game aside, except to keep it in mind for future reference, the aim now is twofold. One, to make use of all existing avenues to manage those already addicted to these highly potent and dangerous medications. Second, to save future generations from succumbing to tainted information and to protect them from falling into the same catastrophic situation.

As a doctor, there are some things I can control and some I can't. I can try, to the best of my ability, to prescribe exactly what a patient needs in terms of pain relief, to track the dosage, to refuse to write another prescription before the previous prescription should have run out, to randomly drug test my patients, and so on. Even with all that, a patient could still buy more of a medication on the black market. Nor can I stop someone from taking an overdose.

These are some of the scenarios that could lead to the misuse of a drug:

1. An elderly person might take his or her medication several times in a short period because of a memory lapse.
2. A patient might misunderstand or misjudge the amount of time it takes a particular medication to "kick in." Thus, when no relief is felt in what that patient feels is a reasonable time, he or she may take another pill under the assumption that more is needed. Methadone, for example, takes a long time to work its way through the system—sometimes as long as twenty-four hours. Even though its effect might be muted, it would still be unsafe, even fatal, to follow the first dose with another pill before the allotted time.
3. A depressed person, living alone, might be more inclined to combine too many pills with alcohol, anxiety medications, and sleeping pills.
4. The same patient, in too much pain to work or even be active, might be tempted to get high on an extra pill out of boredom.

No physician in his or her right mind wants patients to overdose on the drugs he or she prescribes. Besides the emotional toll of contributing to a tragedy, such an event can result in a malpractice suit, serious damage to the doctor's reputation, or even law enforcement scrutiny.

There is a distinct difference between dependence and addiction, as Dr. Scott Fishman explains on his website MDJunction:

> Addiction is a biological and psychological condition that compels a person to satisfy their need for a particular stimulus and to keep satisfying it, no matter what. It is a compulsive behavior that de-

mands more and more drugs, regardless of the consequences that lead to dysfunction. A person who is addicted to opioids has a disease that undermines optimal function and drives one to compulsively use a drug, despite the negative consequences.

The pain patient who is effectively treated with opioids finds life restored—even if he is dependent on them. With the pain muted by stable and steady controlled use of long-acting opioids, a patient can reclaim his life, go back to work, return to family life, and pursue favorite pastimes. Dependence is a physical state that occurs when the lack of a drug causes the body to have a reaction. Physical dependence is solely a physical state indicating that the body has grown so adapted to having the drug present that sudden removal of it will lead to negative consequences such as a withdrawal reaction. This can occur with almost any kind of drug.

A good example of dependence is a heavy coffee drinker's use of caffeine. If you are used to drinking several cups of coffee each day, you soon learn about physical dependence when you miss a day or two. This does not mean you are addicted to the caffeine; it only means your body is surprised not to see what it has come to expect.

In the case of opioids, a certain amount taken every day fills the glass, and no more may be needed or desired. If the medication is removed, the consequences are physical (sweating, running nose, diarrhea, racing heart, or nausea), not psychological.[7]

People who are addicted, on the other hand, often find themselves craving more and more of that substance. In the case of heroin addicts, they eventually reach a point where they no longer seek out the drug to get high but simply to feel normal.

Another dubious term that received considerable attention at the turn of the century was *pseudoaddiction*. The teaching was that when patients are not getting enough medications, usually opioids, they demand additional pain medications, not because of addiction but because of undertreated pain. Since then, there has been considerable discussion and debunking of this myth.

An investigative review searched Medline articles containing the term *pseudoaddiction* to determine its footprint in literature with a focus on how it has been characterized and empirically validated. The authors found "no empirical evidence yet exists to justify a clinical 'diagnosis' of pseudoaddiction. The renaming of pain with a term that essentially means 'fake addiction' and serves to dismiss addiction as part of the clinical differential diagnosis is a construct that is conspicuously and uniquely attached to opioid therapies which are extremely addictive analgesics, among many other effective, evidence-based strategies for analgesia that are far less addictive."[8]

With any drug, close communication between the prescriber and patient is essential. If something isn't working, or isn't working as well as it once did, I need to know about it. Then we can consider either changing the dosage or switching to something else.

The worst thing one can do is to arbitrarily begin gobbling more pills in an effort to regain the former effect. This can be dangerous and even fatal. If a patient does not suffer dangerous or fatal consequences, he or she still may have difficulty obtaining the next prescription early or may lose the privileges of getting the opioid medications altogether because of the breach of contract with the providing physician.

Such situations have given rise to the illegal street practice of "loaning" pills, for a price, to an individual who has run out of them.

Occasionally, I have encountered patients whom my instincts told me not to treat with opioids. There was, for example, a young man who complained of pain from a "hole in his nose." At first, I was puzzled by this, especially given his age, until I discovered that he had been a heavy cocaine user and this habit had actually resulted in perforation of his nasal septum. Given the current legal and law enforcement climate, prescribing drugs for someone with an addictive history is asking for trouble.

It is also a red flag if someone asks me for a specific drug rather than just something to help with their pain. I have had a few patients tell me that if I didn't give them enough of a particular medication, they would "go out and get it on the street."

For the most part, however, those who come to me are there because they want to be freed from their pain. They generally follow my instructions, and they understand when I explain to them that because everyone's body chemistry is different, a medication that might work for one person could be ineffective when given to another. A certain amount of experimentation is essential to performing my job.

Drugs, like guns, can be deadly when used irresponsibly. I find myself most appalled by a teenage practice called *pharming*, in which guests at a party grab handfuls of assorted (and, generally, unknown) pills from a communal bowl. Known colloquially as *trail mix*, these pills come from medicine cabinets. At the very least, there could be some dicey interactions. The worst-case scenario would end in death.

Part of the reason some teenagers, and adults, may abuse and over-dose on medications might be the thought that prescribed drugs by definition cannot be so dangerous. Nothing can be further from the truth—as we have witnessed in the last two decades. Not only can pain medications cause complications, but they can, and do, kill.

In her song "The Living," Natalie Merchant describes alcohol as "my closest of friends; my worst enemy."

As you will see in the next chapter, the same can be said of opioid painkillers. They may be a friend, but they can also take your life.

2

THE OPIOID EPIDEMIC THAT IS KILLING US

The year 2016 was one of the three worst years in the last decade for terrorism-related deaths worldwide. A total of 25,621 people died.[1]

The U.S. government does not track death rates for every drug. However, the National Center for Health Statistics at the Centers for Disease Control and Prevention (CDC) does collect information on many of the more commonly used drugs. In 2016, as many as sixty-four thousand people died from overdose.[2] That means overdose claimed more than twice as many people as terrorism in the same year. The same report shows that there was a 1.6-fold increase in the total number of deaths between 2010 and 2015 involving the use of cocaine, a 4.3-fold increase involving benzodiazepines, a 5.9-fold increase involving heroin and nonmethadone synthetics, and a 6.2-fold increase involving heroin alone. The deaths involving prescription pain relievers, excluding nonmethadone synthetics, rose 1.9-fold from 2002 to 2011.

Let's break that sixty-four thousand number down. That would mean there were 7 deaths an hour and more than 175 deaths per day—a staggering number!

Now let us imagine a scenario where any other epidemic is killing 175 Americans every day. Not only would it be devastating, it would be headline news, 24/7. There would be an overwhelming response from the federal and state governments. We would be using every possible resource, manpower, and funding to tackle it as quickly as possible.

In fact, on October 8, 2017, the federal government did declare the opioid crisis a healthcare emergency. The U.S. Department of Health and Human Services had previously announced that they would declare a much bigger, national emergency under the Stafford Act. That would have made billions in emergency funding available through FEMA's Disaster Relief Fund. However, the Public Health Emergency Fund currently holds only $57,000 as a result of Congress failing to replenish it for several years, according to Dr. Jake Ende of the American College of the Physicians.[3]

How did we get here?

In a report from the CDC:

> Drug overdose deaths in the United States more than tripled from 1999 to 2015. The current epidemic of drug overdoses began in the 1990s, driven by increasing deaths from prescription opioids that paralleled a dramatic increase in the prescribing of such drugs for chronic pain. In 2008, the number of deaths involving prescription opioids exceeded the number of deaths from heroin and cocaine combined. Since 2010, however, the U.S. has also seen sharp increases in deaths from heroin, synthetic opioids such as fentanyl, cocaine, and methamphetamine. In addition to deaths, overdoses from drugs both prescription and illicit are responsible for parallel increasing trends in nonfatal emergency department and hospital admissions. Morbidity and mortality statistics, however, fail to capture the full extent of the problem with substance use disorders in the United States. Survey data indicate that tens of millions of Americans misuse prescription opioids, sedatives, tranquilizers, and stimulants. Others use illicit drugs such as heroin, fentanyl, cocaine, and methamphetamine. Most persons using heroin have had a history of misusing prescription opioids first. The problem with misuse of prescription drugs of various kinds is related to high levels of prescribing of such medications. For example, in 2016 prescribers wrote 66.5 opioid and 25.2 sedative prescriptions for every 100 Americans.[4]

A *Washington Post* report reveals there is a distinct geographic footprint for opioid deaths in 2015. For example, in 2015 there were up to thirty-six deaths per one hundred thousand in New England and the Ohio/Kentucky/West Virginia region. However, the rates were low in Texas, California, and Hawaii. Heroin deaths were highest in New England states like Massachusetts and Connecticut, as opposed to other states like Maine, Vermont, or New Hampshire. The synthetic opioids like fentanyl and tramadol were exclusively an East Coast phenomenon, killing as many as 24.1 per 100,000 in New Hampshire in 2015. Classic drugs like oxycodone and hydrocodone were highest in West Virginia and Utah. The report highlights that many opioid overdose deaths involve multiple substances, either combinations of opioids or opioids in conjunction with substances like alcohol, cocaine, or other drugs.[5]

Josh Katz reports in the *New York Times* that there has been 22 percent increase in opioid-related deaths from the previous year. The largest number was for white males forty-five to fifty-four years old. Part of it might be that homeless veterans are becoming heroin or illicit fentanyl addicts. The report also noted that this is not just a "rural white problem" in Appalachia and New England. According to the article, it appears that "fentanyls are changing the equation: The death rate in Maryland last year outpaced that in both Kentucky and Maine." The steepest increases were in Maryland, Kentucky, and Delaware.[6]

Fentanyl deserves a special mention.

Pharmaceutical fentanyl is a synthetic opioid pain reliever approved for treating severe pain, typically advanced cancer pain.[7] It is fifty to one hundred times more potent than morphine. It is prescribed in the form of transdermal patches or lozenges and can be diverted for misuse and abuse in the United States. However, most recent cases of fentanyl-related harm, overdose, and death in the United States are linked to illegally made fentanyl. It is sold through illegal drug markets for its heroin-like effect. It is often mixed with heroin and/or cocaine as a combination product—with or without the user's knowledge—to increase its euphoric effects.[8]

An analysis on America's state of mind by Medco Health Solutions reveals that up to 26 percent of women and 15 percent of men are using mental health medications. Sixty percent of Americans are taking prescription drugs.

> Overall, the number of Americans on medications used to treat psychological and behavioral disorders has substantially increased since 2001; more than one-in-five adults was on at least one of these medications in 2010, up 22 percent from ten years earlier. Women are far more likely to take a drug to treat a mental health condition than men, with more than a quarter of the adult female population on these drugs in 2010 as compared to 15 percent of men.

Women ages 45 and older showed the highest use of these drugs overall. Surprisingly, it was younger men (ages 20 to 44) who experienced the greatest increase in their numbers, rising 43 percent from 2001 to 2010.

The trends among children are opposite those of adults: boys are the higher utilizers of these medications overall but girls' use has been increasing at a faster rate.[9]

And according to a *JAMA Psychiatry* article: "In 2008, approximately 5.2% of US adults aged 18 to 80 years used benzodiazepines. The percentage who used benzodiazepines increased with age from 2.6% (18–35 years) to 5.4% (36–50 years) to 7.4% (51–64 years) to 8.7% (65–80 years). Benzodiazepine use was nearly twice as prevalent in women as men."[10]

An additional complicating factor is the ingestion of alcohol. Combining alcohol with prescription drugs is a deadly mix.

The implications of mixing potent medications and alcohol are enormous. Frequently, these potentiate each other and lead to serious risks that include respiratory depression and death. This may be a major contributing factor in the mortality numbers we are experiencing as a nation with a current opioid epidemic.

Given that a large number of our population is on one or more medications, the risk of major calamity is not too far away from many of us. When we discuss the percentages of deaths from drugs, we usually think of it as only involving drug addicts in some remote place, far away from us. The reality, and tragedy, is closer than we realize. Given how many of us, or our family members, friends, and relatives, are on just one antidepressant, one sleeping pill, one anxiety medicine, or one opioid. The chances of drug interactions and serious risks are plenty.

I tend to closely study the celebrity deaths from drug overdose. Specifically, I try to figure out what exactly it is that is killing all these young people. Over the years, I have found that very few, if any, died of a single drug overdose. Most of the time it is a deadly combination of multiple medications, frequently mixed with alcohol.

Responding to this major crisis, the CDC issued a new report, titled *CDC Guideline for Prescribing Opioids for Chronic Pain*.[11] It focuses on trying nonopioid medications first, starting low and going slow, and regular follow-ups. The specific guidelines are summarized below:

1. "Nonpharmacologic therapy and nonopioid pharmacologic therapy are preferred for chronic pain. Clinicians should consider opioid therapy only if expected benefits for both pain and function are anticipated to outweigh risks to the patient. If opioids are used, they should be combined with nonpharmacologic therapy and nonopioid pharmacologic therapy, as appropriate."

2. "Before starting opioid therapy for chronic pain, clinicians should establish treatment goals with all patients, including realistic goals for pain and function, and should consider how opioid therapy will be discontinued if benefits do not outweigh risks. Clinicians should continue opioid therapy only if there is clinically meaningful improvement in pain and function that outweighs risks to patient."

3. "Before starting and periodically during opioid therapy, clinicians should discuss with patients known risks and realistic benefits of opioid therapy and patient and clinician responsibilities for managing therapy."

4. "When starting opioid therapy for chronic pain, clinicians should prescribe immediate-release opioids instead of extended-release/long-acting (ER/LA) opioids."

5. "When opioids are started, clinicians should prescribe the lowest effective dosage. Clinicians should use caution when prescribing opioids at any dosage, should carefully reassess evidence of individual benefits and risks when considering increasing dosage to ≥50 morphine milligram equivalents (MME)/day, and should avoid increasing dosage to ≥90 MME/day or carefully justify a decision to titrate dosage to ≥90 MME/day."

6. "Long-term opioid use often begins with treatment of acute pain. When opioids are used for acute pain, clinicians should prescribe the lowest effective dose of immediate-release opioids and should prescribe no greater quantity than needed for the expected duration of pain severe enough to require opioids. Three days or less will often be sufficient; more than seven days will rarely be needed."

7. "Clinicians should evaluate benefits and harms with patients within 1 to 4 weeks of starting opioid therapy for chronic pain or of dose escalation. Clinicians should evaluate benefits and harms of continued therapy with patients every 3 months or more fre-

quently. If benefits do not outweigh harms of continued opioid therapy, clinicians should optimize other therapies and work with patients to taper opioids to lower dosages or to taper and discontinue opioids."

8. "Before starting and periodically during continuation of opioid therapy, clinicians should evaluate risk factors for opioid-related harms. Clinicians should incorporate into the management plan strategies to mitigate risk, including considering offering naloxone when factors that increase risk for opioid overdose, such as history of overdose, history of substance use disorder, higher opioid dosages (≥50 MME/day), or concurrent benzodiazepine use, are present."

9. "Clinicians should review the patient's history of controlled substance prescriptions using state prescription drug monitoring program (PDMP) data to determine whether the patient is receiving opioid dosages or dangerous combinations that put him or her at high risk for overdose. Clinicians should review PDMP data when starting opioid therapy for chronic pain and periodically during opioid therapy for chronic pain, ranging from every prescription to every 3 months."

10. "When prescribing opioids for chronic pain, clinicians should use urine drug testing before starting opioid therapy and consider urine drug testing at least annually to assess for prescribed medications as well as other controlled prescription drugs and illicit drugs."

11. "Clinicians should avoid prescribing opioid pain medication and benzodiazepines concurrently whenever possible."

12. "Clinicians should offer or arrange evidence-based treatment (usually medication-assisted treatment with buprenorphine or methadone in combination with behavioral therapies) for patients with opioid use disorder."[12]

We now also have the ability to manage chronic pain with evidence-based, minimally invasive interventional procedures that include nerve blocks, ablation procedures, and neuromodulation techniques like spinal cord, deep brain, and peripheral nerve stimulation. Add to this a wide selection of safer, nonopioid medications and nerve pain medications. This list includes antidepressants and antiseizure medications, and nonsteroidal anti-inflammatory medications and muscle relaxants, to name a few. In most situations, if these are employed as indicated early in the course of treatment, along with physical therapy and possibly psychological help, there may be few cases that would still require an opioid.

Rightly so, many pain practices have already stopped or greatly reduced writing opioid prescriptions for chronic pain, and others are in the process of doing so.

Let's hope that all of us, as a nation, finally wake up and realize the enormous price we are paying with overdose deaths and do whatever we can to make a better today and a safer tomorrow.

3

ON ADDICTION MANAGEMENT

As a nation, we are reeling under the worst opioid crisis ever. It is killing our young and old in large numbers every day and devastating our communities. There is an urgent need for a major intervention. And we are lagging behind.

The American Society of Addiction Medicine (ASAM), the premier agency involved in the management of addiction in the nation,

> defines addiction as "a primary, chronic disease of brain reward, motivation, memory, and related circuitry," with a "dysfunction in these circuits" being reflected in "an individual pathologically pursuing reward and/or relief by substance use and other behaviors." In this context, the preferred term by ASAM for this serious bio-psycho-social-spiritual illness would be "addiction involving opioid use." ASAM views addiction as a fundamental neurological disorder of "brain reward, motivation, memory, and related circuitry," and recognizes that there are unifying features in all cases of addiction, including substance-related addiction and nonsubstance-related addiction. It is clear that a variety of substances commonly associated with addiction work on specific receptors in the nervous system and on specific neurotransmitter systems. Specific pharmacological agents used in the treatment of addiction exert their effects via their actions on specific receptors. Hence, the medications used in the treatment of addiction have specific efficacy based on their own molecular structure and the particular neurotransmitters affected by that medication. Medications developed for the treatment of addiction involving opioid use may have benefits in the treatment of addic-

tion involving an individual's use of other substances. For instance, naltrexone, which is approved by the U.S. Food and Drug Administration (FDA) for the treatment of opioid dependence using DSM, 4th Edition (DSM-IV) terminology, is also US FDA–approved for the treatment of alcohol dependence as per the DSM-IV guidelines.

The American Society of Addiction Medicine recognizes that research is yet to be done to confirm the specificity of its conceptualization of addiction as a medical and a psychiatric illness. Both the American Medical Association, as noted in various policy and position statements, and the *International Classification of Diseases* (ICD), recognize addiction as both a medical and a psychiatric disorder. ASAM encourages clinicians, researchers, educators, and policy makers to use the term "addiction" regardless of whether the patient's condition at a given point in its natural history seems to more prominently involve opioid use, alcohol use, nicotine use, or engagement in addictive behaviors such as gambling. Given the widespread North American application of the DSM's categorization of disorders, this *Practice Guideline* will, for the sake of brevity and convention, use the term "opioid use disorder."[1]

Not long ago, methadone maintenance used to be the drug of choice for management of addiction. The idea was to provide medications, usually on a daily basis, under supervised conditions in combination with counseling and behavioral modifications. With time, the experts have added newer medications like buprenorphine, a combination of buprenorphine with naloxone (Suboxone), and naltrexone.

There has been added funding for these addiction treatment programs. The recent decision by the federal government to designate opioid addiction as a healthcare emergency, though not sufficient, should bring some additional resources. However, the sheer magnitude of the problem demands a great deal of extensive commitment, resources, and funding to even put a dent in this major epidemic.

According to ASAM, "of the 20.5 million Americans 12 or older that had a substance use disorder in 2015, 2 million had a substance use disorder involving prescription pain relievers and 591,000 had a substance use disorder involving heroin. It is estimated that 23% of individuals who use heroin develop opioid addiction."[2] ASAM reports that "drug overdose is the leading cause of accidental death in the US, with 52,404 lethal drug overdoses in 2015. Opioid addiction is driving this epidemic, with 20,101 overdose deaths related to prescription pain relievers, and 12,990 overdose deaths related to heroin in 2015."[3]

A Blue Cross Blue Shield (BCBS) report states that opioids kill more in any year than those killed "at the peak of the human immunodeficiency virus (HIV) epidemic."[4] "Opioid abuse/overdose is considered a leading cause of shortened life expectancy in the U.S."[5]

That report highlights that the nation's opioid epidemic reflects a complex set of circumstances. The pattern of opioid prescribing—including dose and duration—and the patient's risk factors of age, gender, and condition are major determinants of whether a patient becomes dependent.

A summary of key findings in this report shows that patients filling high-dose opioid prescriptions have a much higher rate of opioid use disorder than those filling low-dose prescriptions. BCBS also reports that from 2010 to 2016, there was a 493 percent increase in opioid use disorder.[6]

The 2016 surgeon general's report *Facing Addiction in America* found that only one in ten people receive specialized treatments to manage their addictions.[7]

In a separate chapter, we have discussed the events that may be linked to the development of this addiction crisis that we are seeing now. A recent analysis[8] titled "Who Is Responsible for the Pain-Pill Epidemic?" illustrates the crisis well and is worth a read.

For those already addicted to opioids and, consequently, to their serious risks, an Office-Based Opioid Treatment (OBOT) is currently considered the most reasonable management option. The principles of this approach include the following:

1. The choice of available treatment options for addiction involving opioid use should be a shared decision between clinician and patient.
2. Clinicians should consider the patient's preferences, past treatment history, and treatment setting when deciding between the use of methadone, buprenorphine, and naltrexone in the treatment of addiction involving opioid use. . . .
3. The venue in which treatment is provided is as important as the specific medication selected. Opioid treatment programs (OTPs) offer daily supervised dosing of methadone, and increasingly of buprenorphine. . . .

4. OBOT may not be suitable for patients with active alcohol use disorder or sedative, hypnotic, or anxiolytic use disorder (or who are in the treatment of addiction involving the use of alcohol or other sedative drugs, including benzodiazepines or benzodiazepine receptor agonists). . . .

5. Methadone is recommended for patients who may benefit from daily dosing and supervision in an OTP, or for patients for whom buprenorphine for the treatment of opioid use disorder has been used unsuccessfully in an OTP or OBOT setting.

6. Oral naltrexone for the treatment of opioid use disorder is often adversely affected by poor medication adherence. Clinicians should reserve its use for patients who would be able to comply with special techniques to enhance their adherence, for example, observed dosing. Extended release injectable naltrexone reduces, but does not eliminate, issues with medication adherence.

In an extensive analysis, the National Institute on Drug Abuse/National Institutes of Health (NIH) found:

Like other chronic diseases, addiction can be managed successfully. Treatment enables people to counteract addiction's powerful disruptive effects on the brain and behavior and to regain control of their lives. The chronic nature of the disease means that relapsing to drug abuse is not only possible but also likely, with symptom recurrence rates similar to those for other well-characterized chronic medical illnesses—such as diabetes, hypertension, and asthma that also have both physiological and behavioral components.

Unfortunately, when relapse occurs many deem treatment a failure. This is not the case: Successful treatment for addiction typically requires continual evaluation and modification as appropriate, similar to the approach taken for other chronic diseases. For example, when a patient is receiving active treatment for hypertension and symptoms decrease, treatment is deemed successful, even though symptoms may recur when treatment is discontinued. For the addicted individual, lapses to drug abuse do not indicate failure—rather, they signify that treatment needs to be reinstated or adjusted, or that alternate treatment is needed.[9]

The report lists a relapse rate of 40–60 percent for drug addiction, as compared to 50 percent for diabetes and up to 70 percent for asthma.

Further, analysis looks at if the drug addiction treatment is worth its cost:

> Substance abuse costs our Nation over $600 billion annually and treatment can help reduce these costs. Drug addiction treatment has been shown to reduce associated health and social costs by far more than the cost of the treatment itself. Treatment is also much less expensive than its alternatives, such as incarcerating addicted persons. For example, the average cost for 1 full year of methadone maintenance treatment is approximately $4,700 per patient, whereas 1 full year of imprisonment costs approximately $24,000 per person.
>
> The National Institute on Drug Abuse/NIH report referenced above also observes that every dollar invested in addiction treatment programs yields a return of between $4 and $7 in reduced drug-related crime, criminal justice costs, and theft. When savings related to healthcare are included, total savings can exceed costs by a ratio of 12 to 1. Major savings to the individual and to society also stem from fewer interpersonal conflicts; greater workplace productivity; and fewer drug-related accidents, including overdoses and deaths.[10]

The first step to breaking the shell of addiction is to realize and admit that one has a problem. There should be no attempt at making excuses or dredging up the justifications.

As Jen Knox, author of *The Glass City and Other Stories*, is quoted as saying, "An intelligent person can rationalize anything, a wise person doesn't try."[11]

4

THE MYSTERY OF PAIN

Sooner or later, most of what afflicts the human body begins to make sense.

Over the centuries, we gradually learned about germs, viruses, new ways of healing, and the connection between cleanliness and health. We learned that we were often responsible for our own physical ills, in a myriad of ways. Ultimately, we came to realize that through medication and lifestyle changes, we could actually alter what was happening to our bodies.

In many cases, it was as simple as cause and effect. Too little exercise and too much fatty food equal clogged arteries and a potential heart attack or stroke. Too much sugar may predispose one to, or worsen, diabetes. Inhaling smoke into one's lungs can irritate them to the point of disease. One at a time, these insights were bestowed upon the healers, often through much trial and error.

Of course, there have always been mysteries to unravel. Cancer, a Trojan horse that attacked from within, was a malevolent and virtually unsolvable cipher for generations of physicians. Now that the causes have become known for some types of cancer, treatment strategies are evolving. Meanwhile, the subtleties of diabetes, HIV/AIDS, Alzheimer's disease, and a host of other enemies of health remain to be sorted out.

The earliest humans could not have deduced that pain comes from messages sent from nerve endings to receptors in the brain, but they were no doubt well aware that being struck by a club or falling down on the rock floor of a cave hurt. And that sometimes the hurt didn't go away.

Pain is a basic fact of life, an unwanted companion to humanity since before we began walking upright.

Still, late twentieth- and early twenty-first-century research on pain has created a curious dichotomy. The more we learn about acute pain, the more illogical its evil twin, chronic pain, becomes.

In the case of acute pain, communications from the nerves generally fly straight and true to the brain: "We have a situation here!" Their purpose is to alert us to injury and illness. They are on our side.

Chronic pain, on the other hand, can act like a malfunctioning GPS device. Its messages can sometimes wander awry, sending the alarm to somewhere in Kansas instead of Chicago. Sometimes the message gets caught in a ceaseless viral loop, declaring the presence of pain over and over again.

Even stranger, the stridency of the alarm isn't always connected to the damage that triggered it. Some patients with reflex sympathetic dystrophy or postherpetic neuralgia find their torment unleashed not from a broken bone or severe trauma but by reaching down to pick up a book or twisting slightly while exiting a car. For them, the punishment far exceeds the crime.

In her brilliant memoir and examination of chronic pain, *The Pain Chronicles*, Melanie Thernstrom writes: "Persistent pain has the opaque quality of a torturer who seems to taunt us toward imagining that there is an answer that would stop the next blow. But whatever we come up with does not suffice."[1]

From Wikipedia to the most complex medical textbook, the same sentence appears over and over: "There is no cure for chronic pain."

I cannot agree with that unequivocally, because I have occasionally seen chronic pain disappear. And if that happens, something made it go away.

Perhaps a more accurate statement would be: "There is no universal cure for chronic pain."

From the perspective of treatment, most diseases and conditions leave essentially the same footprint upon their victims. There are certainly variables: how far advanced the ailment, how large the tumor, how strong the constitution of the patient, and so on. Physicians dealing with lung cancer, hepatitis, whooping cough, or a host of other familiar afflictions tend to start out with strategies from the same playbook.

The nature of chronic pain is full of mysteries. Why would the same injury that would heal in two weeks for one person condemn another to a lifetime of discomfort or even agony? Is it genetic? A malfunction of the pain receptors? A problem with the brain? We're still not sure. There is no answer yet that will satisfy the torturer.

In a paper titled "Problems in the Differential Diagnosis of Chronic Pain," physician and University of Michigan professor Kenneth L. Casey writes:

> There seems to be general agreement that a disturbance of input to the central nervous system can result in long-term central changes that may alter the excitability of central neurons that transmit nociceptive information.
>
> These central anatomical and physiological changes may persist and sustain the painful state at least as long as the pathological condition continues in the periphery. However, there is no evidence, to my knowledge, that chronic pain itself induces a clinically detectable patho-physiological state, in central neurons, that allows pain to continue in the absence of any organic pathology.[2]

Rough translation: There are times when chronic pain makes no sense.

Medical science has come rather late to this puzzle for a very basic reason. Before it could be treated, chronic pain first had to be believed in.

The recognition of chronic pain as a distinct, stand-alone condition came only after three long-held beliefs were refuted:

1. Chronic pain is not a separate entity but merely a symptom of other ailments.
2. Chronic pain is merely a function of aging, the normal "aches and pains" inevitable for a high-mileage body.
3. With some patients, chronic pain is a creature of the imagination. They hurt because they think they do, as if through some self-imposed voodoo.

The problem, of course, is that no one has yet invented a pain meter. Health professionals can attach various devices to their patients that will register and calibrate blood pressure, temperature, brain waves, and a host of other bodily functions but not how much pain is being experienced.

Every school-hating kid knows this.

"I don't feel good," they tell their mothers as the yellow bus makes its rounds. "I've got a stomachache."

Attached is the unspoken challenge: "Prove that I don't."

Because chronic pain essentially makes no medical sense, the temptation was always to dismiss it. In recent years, however, doctors have learned some ways to use standard instruments to test some of the peripheral effects of pain: increased blood pressure, quickened heartbeat, reactions to touch, temperature changes, and so on.

Back to Dr. Casey:

> Pain is a subjective experience, and determination of its presence relies entirely upon the report of the individual. The best that can be done with present methods is to systematically consider all possible sources of pathological input that may result in the perception of pain. The diagnostic procedures must be performed with minimal risk to the patient and within the bounds of sound clinical judgment. If no objective pathologic site can be identified, it is important to determine if the patient's psychological profile, as shown by modern testing methods, suggests that the patient's complaints of pain may bear little or no relation to the presence of demonstrable tissue pathology.[3]

To be sure, skeptics remain. Fibromyalgia, a condition that disproportionately affects women, has been a particular target. One of its most vocal nonbelievers in the medical community is Wichita rheumatologist Fred Wolfe.

"We've taken stress, psychosocial distress and pain and the ordinary life experiences people have and turned them into something they're not—a physical illness," Wolfe has said.[4]

Increasingly, however, skeptics like Fred Wolfe appear to be sinking further into the minority. The pharmaceutical industry, which always keeps its antennas raised for a new dragon to slay, has apparently decided that fibromyalgia has reached critical mass. Along with the Three Horsemen of baby boomer nightmares: heart disease, diabetes, and Alzheimer's.

According to a 2009 Associated Press article by Matthew Perrone:

Two drug makers spent hundreds of millions of dollars last year to raise awareness of a murky illness, helping boost sales of pills recently approved as treatments and drowning out unresolved questions—including whether it's a real disease or not.

Key components in the industry-funded buzz over the pain-and-fatigue ailment fibromyalgia are grants—more than $6 million donated by drug-makers Eli Lilly and Pfizer in the first three quarters of 2008—to nonprofit groups for medical conferences and educational campaigns, an Associated Press analysis found.

That's more than they gave for more accepted ailments, such as diabetes and Alzheimer's. Among grants tied to scientific diseases, fibromyalgia ranked third for each company, behind only cancer and AIDS for Pfizer and cancer and depression for Lilly.[5]

Thus, fibromyalgia, often disrespected and dismissed when it was called chronic fatigue syndrome, has broken through the wall of disbelief that surrounded it and taken its place in the pantheon of high-profile targets for Big Pharma.

Certainly, every legitimate drug on the market for any condition is quickly outnumbered by Internet pretenders. Alternative treatments spring up, ranging from cutting-edge possibilities to overt medicine-show hoaxes. Still, at the end of the day (often a painful day for chronic pain sufferers), the pills have to work. A fraud can only be perpetuated for so long on a hurting person.

In 2008, the *New York Times* brewed its own storm of controversy with an article on the FDA's approval of Lyrica for fibromyalgia.

The headline was part of the problem. It read "Drug Approved: Is Disease Real?"

The story continued in the same vein:

Advocacy groups and doctors who treat fibromyalgia estimate that 2 to 4 percent of adult Americans, as many as 10 million people, suffer from the disorder.

Those figures are sharply disputed by those doctors who do not consider fibromyalgia a medically recognizable illness and who say that diagnosing the condition actually worsens suffering by causing patients to obsess over aches that other people simply tolerate. Further, they warn that Lyrica's side effects, which include severe weight gain, dizziness and edema, are very real, even if fibromyalgia is not.[6]

However, the dispute over fibromyalgia doesn't take into account other chronic pain ailments such as reflex sympathetic dystrophy (RSD), which can cause excruciating pain in the affected limb. Or a vicious post-shingles syndrome known as postherpetic neuralgia, which has driven people to suicide.

Meanwhile, doctors continue to struggle with diagnoses. Physicians like myself who embrace the concept of chronic pain have come to believe, in some cases, that sometimes the cause can be of secondary importance. Our goal must be to stop—or at least moderate—the patient's pain, regardless of its origin.

Often, though, many of the "players" in a patient's care demand a specific diagnosis. The patient wants to know what is wrong. The insurance company wants to know how this claim fits into its system of coverage.

In many conditions that fall in the spectrum of chronic pain, such as fibromyalgia and complex regional pain syndrome (CRPS), there may not be positive objective laboratory, radiological, or electrodiagnostic test results. Yet it is important to make what we in the medical community call a "provisional diagnosis" based on a thorough history and detailed examination. This lays down the most plausible explanation and future course for the workup and therapeutic planning. This also gives the patient the benefit of understanding the factors that may be resulting in the symptoms he or she perceives.

In other words, the best that can be done is to determine what is not afflicting the patient. Thus, we frequently arrive at diagnosis by default.

Nevertheless, this is one of medicine's most exciting new frontiers. Across the medical spectrum, weapons are being mobilized against this new threat: newer antineuropathic drugs like antiseizure drugs and antidepressant drugs, nerve blocks, ablation procedures, and peripheral, spinal, and brain-modulating implants. If the brain can play such a prominent role in pain perception, what other secrets or unknown powers might it be hiding?

In her review of Melanie Thernstrom's book, writer Alice Sebold called the treatment of chronic pain "the Wild West of medicine."[7]

As a practicing pain doctor, there's nowhere I would rather be.

5

THE COMPLEX NATURE OF CHRONIC PAIN

Pain is God's midwife, that helps some virtue into existence.

—Henry Ward Beecher

Of all the common denominators of human existence, pain is perhaps the most universal.

It surrounds us like air, never more than a nerve ending away. It announces its presence within and without our bodies, sometimes almost unnoticeable, sometimes excruciating. It is present at our birth and often at our death.

The avoidance of pain has always dictated much of human behavior, yet there are times when seeking it out—for example, on the battlefield—is seen as the epitome of nobility.

In most instances, pain is our ally, our early alert system. If there was no pain to warn of a torn knee ligament, for example, the knee's owner might continue to walk or run on it and do even more grievous damage. It is pain that tells us to yank our hand off a hot stove or to rush to the emergency room to be checked out for chest discomfort.

Those sudden alarms fall under the category of acute pain and are generally not within the realm of the pain specialist. An obvious injury to tissue or organs is treated in emergency rooms, by general practitioners, or by other types of specialists, such as orthopedists. In the case of "good outcomes," as we like to say, pain can be relieved of its duty and sent back to its guard post.

What those in my field grapple with every working day is the rogue pain or chronic pain. Chronic pain is, for reasons still largely unexplained, pain that refuses to go away.

In a broad sense, the way we register pain is somewhat like the way my family summoned the doctor back in Kashmir. The difference, of course, is that this communication is measured in milliseconds rather than hours.

Nevertheless, the process is essentially the same. Initially, it is determined that something potentially unpleasant is happening in some part of the body. Riding the superhighway of the spinal cord, specially adapted nerve fibers scurry to carry this disturbing news to the brain, specifically the limbic region and the prefrontal cortex.

En route, these messages are evaluated and, in an area of the nervous system called the dorsal horn, amplified. You might think of the dorsal horn as the nervous system's version of a radio dispatch center.

The brain then collects the data and passes instructions back to the initial location, and we experience that sensation we call pain. The time lapse between the stubbed toe and the "ouch!" is so fleeting that we don't even notice it, making the injury and the resultant pain seem simultaneous. This is the fast track of pain response.

At the same time, however, a slower channel can follow the initial sensation with a dull, nagging pain, the kind you might feel in your stubbed toe around bedtime, hours later.

Normally, the early warning system against pain is not only efficient but virtually omnipresent. The first sentinels, the nociceptors, are located anywhere pain can occur; virtually anywhere in the body except, oddly enough, the tissue of the brain. They are attached to the ends of sensory nerves and respond to any sort of tissue damage or potential tissue damage (like a heat source drawing uncomfortably close). That response is passed along by the aforementioned nerve fibers.

Try to find a spot anywhere on your body that won't register a pinprick—you can't! The vigilant army of nociceptors has you covered.

There are exceptions to this, of course, and they tend to prove the rule about how pain travels. An Oregon diabetic with no feeling in his feet woke up one day in 2011 to find that his dog had eaten several of his toes (a veterinarian theorized that the dog was trying to help by removing a source of gangrene). A person with normal sensitivity would have been jolted awake with the first bite, but in this case the spinal cord superhighway was blocked somewhere along its path.

In his science fiction novel *The Fall of Hyperion*, Dan Simmons wrote: "Pain has a structure. It has a floor plan. It has designs more intricate than a chambered nautilus."[1]

True enough. The more scientists research the many-chambered process through which we feel pain, the more complicated it becomes. As early as 1965, in an article of *Science* magazine, Ronald Melzack and Patrick Wall introduced a "pain gate" theory. This theory proposes that there are actually two types of messengers contacting the brain, transmission cells and inhibitory cells. The function of the former is to open the gate and allow two-way travel of pain impulses. The latter, the inhibitory cells, are programmed to moderate pain and close the gate.

In other words, if you bang your elbow on a hard object, the transmission cells go berserk. But when you rub your elbow, making it feel better, the inhibitory cells chime in with "Wait a minute, it's not that bad."

Again, acute pain is the prompt and immediate reminder that something is wrong. Chronic pain is the helpful friend who has outstayed his welcome and become a nag. It can hide in the labyrinth of nerve endings that make up Simmons's "chambered nautilus," popping up in unlikely places, far removed from its actual source. At its worst, it can be almost impossible to eradicate.

In his book, *Self-Management of Chronic Pain: Patient Handbook*, Dr. Richard W. Hanson writes:

> A large part of this apparent puzzle (of chronic pain) . . . results from a failure to understand the active role played by the brain in pain perception. According to this view, the brain is simply a passive receiver that picks up pain signals that are generated and transmitted directly from the site of the injury. In other words, the brain is seen to work something like a telephone or radio receiver that accurately reproduces whatever messages are sent to it.
>
> In reality, the brain is not simply a passive receiver, nor is the spinal cord a passive conveyor of pain messages originating in some injured part of the body. Rather, both of these central nervous system structures play an active role in modifying the pain messages that are ultimately registered in the brain. Furthermore, the brain serves as both a receiver and an active transmitter. It can transmit

signals that block the experience of pain. It can also significantly magnify the experience of pain out of proportion to the original injury, or it can even generate signals which lead a person to experience pain in a part of the body that is not actually injured.[2]

Murphy's Law is not to be found in any medical textbooks, but it may have some bearing here. Anyone who works in technology comes to realize that the more wondrous and complicated a piece of machinery or electronic apparatus may be, the more things can go wrong. It's not hard to imagine, then, how a system through which the brain not only receives but interprets pain signals, dispenses endorphins and other pain-easing chemicals like an in-house druggist, and even, somehow, instinctively "knows" how serious an injury might be—all in the space of nanoseconds—might be fair game for Mr. Murphy.

For example, researchers believe that the body's early warning system sometimes becomes stuck. Melanie Thernstrom, a chronic pain sufferer herself, provides this vivid metaphorical description:

> Imagine a home security alarm system that is first triggered by a cat, then a breeze, and then, for no reason, begins to ring randomly or continuously. As it continues to ring, it triggers other noises in the house: the radio and television start to blare; the oven timer dings; the doorbell buzzes repeatedly; and the phone rings maniacally even though no one has placed a call. This is neuropathic pain.[3]

In other cases, as described in "Pain Perception—the Dana Guide," the problems lie not with the brain or the spinal cord gates and pathways but with an individual nerve or group of nerves:

> If significant tissue damage has occurred, or if there has been a prolonged or particular intense activation of a primary . . . nociceptor, it will become sensitized. Sensitized nociceptors can be activated by modern stimuli that normally don't produce pain. One common example of sensitized nociceptors is the agony produced by bath or shower water on sensitized skin.[4]

Neuropathic pain is the flip side of nociceptive pain, a much more open-and-shut proposition. And it raises an intriguing philosophical and medical question: What, exactly, is pain?

Is pain the initial impulse that travels to the brain, or is it our reaction when that message comes bouncing back like a satellite signal? What about the man with the foot-eating dog? Was pain involved in his injury, or was it the neurological version of the tree falling in the forest?

Some people have been known to lose limbs or suffer major trauma and feel no immediate pain at all—a tribute to the body's ability to respond to massive trauma with a rush of self-generated pain killers. Years later, however, the same person may experience significant discomfort from the site of an arm or leg long gone.

The phenomenon known as *phantom limb pain* remains baffling, a curious link between imagination and bodily function. If the brain can tell us that we are in pain from something that no longer exists, could it also be tricked into other inappropriate but potentially useful responses? To pay a quick visit to the dark side, what if torturers could merely suggest to their victims that they are being painfully tortured, thus leaving no evidence behind?

It is equally possible, of course, that phantom limb syndrome (PLS) stems from the remnants of nerves that have been partially amputated but not disconnected. Even this theory, however, defies clinical substantiation.

Increasingly, pain bedevils not only physicians but lawyers, insurance companies, and government agencies. As the mind-body connection emerges as more real and more complex, the actual presence of pain becomes more elusive. Someday, perhaps, we might be able to hook up a device to a person who claims to be in pain and register not only the veracity of his or her statement but the severity of the hurt. Not yet.

Still, there is no denying that the mind plays a key role in how pain is perceived. Studies have shown that a dental patient expecting a procedure to be extremely painful will often invite that pain into his or her mouth. Similarly, with chronic pain patients, pain becomes so much a part of their lives—a path grooved so deeply into the brain—that it is accepted as their daily reality.

The key to truly effective treatment is finding an off switch. If the network of nerve fibers can turn on the body's reaction to pain, there should be a way to turn it off.

Scientists have discovered that certain chemicals—everything from globulin to potassium to histamine to various acids—trigger a response from the nociceptors. If the same chemicals are injected in very small doses, they generally cause immediate pain.

Are these chemicals, then, the physical manifestation of pain? Or are they only its enablers? And by what mechanism are they secreted when pain threatens?

According to the most commonly quoted count, one in three Americans suffers from some form of chronic pain. Given the nature of Western society, however, many of those affected are psychologically ill equipped to deal with the pain. The myriad TV ads for pain relievers almost always imply a speedy relief from discomfort, a change immediately evident in the sufferer's body language and facial expression. The reality is that most pain medicines merely pull a temporary shroud over the hurt without dealing with the root cause.

As a society, we are not patient. When something hurts, we want and expect that unpleasant feeling to go away as quickly as possible. And when the normal cause and effect breaks down, it jolts our mental equilibrium.

Physicians often feel the backlash of this. We all hate to receive that phone call in which a strained voice on the other end tells us: "It *still* hurts. What do I do?"

Often that's a tough question.

Acute pain is much easier to deal with. An abscessed tooth can be pulled. A broken leg can be set. In these instances, medication serves the useful function of holding the worst of the discomfort at bay until natural healing takes over.

But what if that healing never comes? What if the pain lasts for months or even years, long after the original injury or condition has been declared "fixed"?

Patients referred to pain specialists are usually at this point—and despite all our specialized knowledge, we often find ourselves groping in the dark. Even a relevant description of an individual's pain can be elusive. It can be sharp, dull, or somewhere in between. It can be a pins-and-needles feeling or a stabbing assault. It can be constant or intermittent. It can be all of those things at different times.

Moreover, pain cannot be quantified in any meaningful way. The Mayo Clinic, among others, uses a 1–10 point system, with 0–1 being no pain, 2–3 mild pain, 4–5 moderate pain, 6–7 severe pain, 8–9 intense pain, and 10 unbearable pain. The problem is, unlike body temperature or blood pressure, these numbers are subjective and individualized. What is a 2 pain to one patient might be a 7 to someone else.

On many occasions, I have performed the same surgical procedure on two different patients on the same day. One patient appears to be in extreme discomfort and asks for relief from his pain, the stronger the better. The other patient stoically endures the procedure with no apparent distress and no medication.

Just as beauty is in the eye of the beholder, pain is often in the nervous system of the afflicted. We have learned that pain tolerance varies widely from patient to patient, and the basic questions "Does this hurt?" and "How does it hurt?" might receive a multitude of answers.

Most physicians consider any pain that persists for more than six months to be chronic. Others push that dividing line up to four months or even three. It often depends on the condition itself. A bone injury will, for example, take longer to heal than one to soft tissue. If a patient is an eighty-five-year-old with chronic arthritis, I would prescribe pain medication differently than I might for a younger person with a sports injury.

We take our pain to doctors and hospitals for two primary reasons: (1) to find out what's causing it and (2) to make it stop. In some cases, the first can be as important as the second.

Pain of unknown origin activates not only our nerves but our psyches. We worry. Someone with persistent severe headaches might start thinking: "What if I have a brain tumor?" or "Is this going to hurt me forever?"

One of my first tasks, then, is to try and rule out some of the more disturbing possibilities. I might run an MRI, a brain scan. Often the very knowledge that a person's pain is not necessarily leading him or her down a final path is enough to make that person feel better.

But not always. I have heard of those who committed suicide not from incurable cancer or Alzheimer's disease but from the unremitting bite of post-shingles complications or some other non–life threatening (yet painful) malady. After months or years of discomfort, the person simply decides he or she is unwilling to continue a torturous life without relief.

Generally, we can group chronic pain into one of two categories— nociceptive or neuropathic. The former originates in the skeletal system, muscles, tissues, or organs; the latter in the nerves themselves.

Perhaps the best-known incidence of the latter is the increasingly high-profile condition of fibromyalgia. Another common manifestation is reflex sympathetic dystrophy (RSD).

In a sense, every pain is neuropathic in that it is transmitted through the nerves. The good news in the field of pain is that symptoms that were once deemed imagined have in recent years been given names. Research into fibromyalgia and RSD (aka complex regional pain syndrome or CRPS) has accelerated, and medications are beginning to emerge from the pharmacological pipeline.

Alas, there is still no cure for many neuropathic disorders. When acute pain mutates into chronic, the focus often must shift from solving the medical problem to ensuring the function of the patient.

Chronic pain affects not only bodies but families and careers. Human resource departments and insurance companies can, like the chronic pain patients themselves, become impatient. As missed work time multiplies, employers fret that a hole is developing in their operational flow chart. The term *malingering* might be whispered, if not actively voiced. Spouses, children, and friends can grow weary of hearing the same complaints over and over with no apparent end in sight.

All of these things are major challenges for the pain doctor. He or she must, by definition, become an expert in four fields: neurology, psychiatry, anesthesiology, and rehabilitative medicine. Maybe that's why there are only 4,014 of us currently practicing in the United States compared to the current U.S. population of 300 million people.[5]

Nevertheless, there is a certain stark wonder to be seen not only in the body's complicated reaction to painful stimuli but in the times when the nerve/brain system malfunctions. In a sense, there is a twisted sort of nobility to the tiny gatekeepers that continue to stand watch even in what would seem the absence of obvious trauma. They are wrong, but they are steadfast. In their primitive way, they are relying on faith.

In many cases, those of us who seek to disconnect them are, too.

6

THE CULTURE OF PAIN

Most medical problems are ethnically and culturally neutral. Flu is flu, a fracture is a fracture, and cancer is cancer, whether the patient lives in Colombia or South Carolina.

However, with chronic pain patients, and those who administer their care, outside factors often enter the equation. Our upbringing, genetics, gender, race, and religion can all affect how we perceive, cope with, and, for providers, manage pain. Unwittingly, we think and act based on preformed ideas.

This reminds me of my niece, a life coach, who's first question to her clients often is: "Whose program are you running?"

A young, Middle Eastern man reported to the emergency room (ER) at the University of Virginia a few years back with chronic pain. During evaluation by an ER doctor, the patient seemed to describe his pain as "killing." As can happen when there is a language barrier, leading to the intended meaning being "lost in translation," the ER doctor felt that the patient said that he would kill himself because of the pain. He called a psychiatry consult and the patient was involuntarily admitted in order to watch him for suicidal ideation. A friend of mine who worked in psychiatry as a physician and spoke the patient's language realized that the patient had only used the word *killing* in Arabic as an analogy to describe his extreme pain. In fact, he started laughing when he realized what had happened. He assured my physician friend that he had no intentions of harming himself and was only illustrating the extent of his chronic suffering.

In addition to language and cultural variations, as illustrated above, perhaps the other most recognizable variable has to do with males and females and how they are raised. In many cultures, male children are taught that pain is to be borne stoically, without tears or complaints. Little girls are usually granted more leeway.

That is not to say that some men aren't demonstrative about pain and some women aren't silent sufferers. I would just argue that these are some typical parameters laid down by society early in life.

As someone born in Kashmir and living in the United States, I have long realized that the Eastern model of reacting to chronic pain is different in many respects from that in the West. For one thing, the culture of machismo is stronger, although gender differences are arguably universal. In an article in the *Los Angeles Times* titled "The Arab version of Machismo Plays an Illicit Role in Mideast Showdown," Nick Williams notes that "in the Arab world, the notion of face is rooted in the ancient traditions of Bedouin honor and the need to protect the family or tribe. Some historians argue that *machismo* was born in these deserts, delivered to Spain in the Arab conquests and transferred to Latin America by the Spanish."[1] Also, the influence of religion is more pervasive.

This is especially true in the Hindu faith. In her article "Pain and Suffering as Viewed by the Hindu Religion," Sarah Whitman of Drexel University's Department of Psychology explains:

> Suffering, both mental and physical, is thought to be part of the unfolding of karma and is the consequence of past inappropriate action (mental, verbal, or physical) that occurred in either one's current life or in a past life. It is not seen as punishment but as a natural consequence of the moral laws of the universe in response to past negative behavior. Hindu traditions promote coping with suffering by accepting it as a just consequence and understanding that suffering is not random. If a Hindu were to ask, "why me?" or feel her circumstances were "not fair," a response would be that her current situation is the exactly correct situation for her to be in, given her soul's previous action. Experiencing current suffering also satisfies the debt incurred for past negative behavior.[2]

Needless to say, this belief could potentially be problematic for the doctor-patient relationship. If the patient were to feel that it was his

duty to suffer, guiding him along any path of treatment might be difficult. Fortunately, Whitman goes on to say, this is usually not the case.

> For Hindus, a first potential challenge may be the feeling of passivity
> or fatalism that may arise because of karma. A patient can feel hope-
> less or unable to change things because he feels that things are fixed
> by karma. Hindu traditions counter this by saying that a person can
> start in the present moment and go forward, living his life in a posi-
> tive way by following dharma. If a patient currently experiences pain,
> change can occur by attending to present appropriate action. If one's
> present state is a consequence of what has gone before, the urgency
> of responsible and appropriate action becomes greater.[3]

Buddhists, meanwhile, are trained to take an interior view of pain,
looking at it as dispassionately as possible. Darlene Cohen, a San Fran-
cisco–based Buddhist and writer, vividly described her struggle with
chronic arthritis in her article "Mindfulness and Pain":

> Here's where meditation and mindfulness come in. Fully inhabiting
> my body, despite its devastation, attentive to every little sensation,
> allowed me to pay close attention to its latent possibilities when they
> appeared. I lived a half-block from the San Francisco Zen Center
> when I was just beginning to be able to take walks again, and I used
> to try to go to dinner there once a week as a treat to myself. Eating a
> good vegetarian meal with other people.
>   Traveling that half-block was my own personal triathlon: walking
> downhill to the front of the building; climbing the stairs, and knock-
> ing on the door with my weak hand. Sometimes I would make it all
> the way to the steps and not be able to go up them. So I would have
> to strain all the way back up the hill to my apartment. I asked myself,
> what is it about my walking that is so tiring? What I called "walking"
> was the part of the step when my foot met the sidewalk. From the
> point of view of the joints, that is the most stressful component of
> walking. The joints get a rest when the foot is in the air, just before it
> strikes the pavement. I found that by focusing on the foot that was in
> the air instead of the foot that was striking the pavement, my stamina
> increased enormously.
>   After making this observation, I never again failed to climb the
> steps to knock on the front door of the Zen Center.[4]

The prominent religion in Kashmir is Islam. In her exhaustive video titled *In Search of a Muslim Pain Principle*, Alcira Molina-Ali arrived at the conclusion that the Muslim attitude toward chronic pain is more self-fulfilling than self-destructive. Like Christians and Jews, Muslims look to their god for healing but are taught to accept divine wisdom if that healing doesn't come.

"Seek treatment for your disease," Muhammad told his disciples. "Allah has not created a disease for which he has not prescribed a cure."[5]

Also, like Christianity and Judaism, Islam is a highly diverse religion, ranging from the rather harsh interpretation practiced in Saudi Arabia to the gentler and more secular Sufi strain.

Because of this, Islam presents a range of cultural differences—often unrelated to religion—to the medical profession. Muslim women, for example, tend to be extremely modest and uncomfortable undressing in front of male doctors.

In the United States, I practice pain medicine within a primarily Christian context. The problem here, at times, is that a devout Christian's fervent belief that God will heal him or her may lead to depression and a sense of failure if that does not occur. Chronic pain, all too often, defies a happy ending.

Generally, however, the differences observed in race, gender, and religion have more to do with the reaction to pain than how the actual pain is perceived. In her study "Pain and Race/Ethnicity," written for the National Pain Foundation, Elisa Martinez observed:

> Pain intensity does not appear to differ across racial groups. That is, the amount of pain—high or low—does not differ. The main differences between African Americans and whites were the differences in their emotional and psychological responses to pain. Pain was more unpleasant and affected the everyday lives of African Americans more than it did white patients.[6]

Martinez went on to list possible reasons for this:

1. Limited access to care and/or quality of care. Because more African Americans have lower income levels and no health insurance, their ability to find quality care might be prevented by their economic status.

2. African-Americans and other minority groups have more distrust of the health care system and their physicians.

3. Some research has shown that African-Americans with pain are more likely to blame themselves for that pain. Also, the fear that pain may prevent one's ability to work may prevent them from seeking treatment.[7]

Of course, this hypothesis is flawed when applied to African Americans in general. While Martinez's theory might fit a warehouse worker or dishwasher who happened to be African American, it would probably not apply to someone of the same ethnicity who was a college professor or attorney—or a doctor.

As it turns out, according to the paper "Culture and Pain" produced by the International Association for the Study of Pain, the endless variety of individual human beings often trumps any effort to conveniently pigeonhole cultural or ethnic groups.

> There are differences within cultural and ethnic groups as well as between them. Several factors affect how closely an individual identifies with his or her ethnic or cultural group. These include gender, age, generation, level of acculturation, socioeconomic status (including income, occupation, and education), level of ties to the mother country, primary language spoken at home, degree of isolation of the individual, and residence in neighborhoods made up of one's ethnic group. These factors may mediate the relationship between ethnic background and pain. For example, only female Italian American outpatients older than 60 tended to report pain more than Anglo-American patients.
>
> Similarly, Neumann and Buskila found that only the older subjects showed significant differences in pain perception in two groups (70 Sephardic and 30 Ashkenazic) of female Israeli patients with fibromyalgia. Lipton and Marbach, using a 35-item scale to measure patients' pain experience, found no significant differences between black, Irish, Italian, Jewish, and Puerto Rican facial pain patients. They did, however, find interethnic differences in emotionality (stoicism versus expressiveness) in response to pain and in pain's interference with daily functioning. In addition, they found that degree of medical acculturation for black patients, degree of social assimilation for Irish patients, duration of pain for Italian patients, and level of psychological distress for Jewish and Puerto Rican patients mediated the pain responses of these groups.[8]

More recently, there has been a plethora of new research that has tried to determine if any genetic components are a significant factor in perception, reaction, and, possibly, maintenance of pain. Here are just a few examples to illustrate the point.

A study of genetic variance in pain perception

> demonstrated (i) a large degree of genetically-determined variability in sensitivity to painful stimuli, (ii) sensitivity to thermal stimuli (hot-plate) is genetically unrelated to sensitivity to chemical (acetic acid) stimuli, (iii) the mechanism by which morphine produces its antinociceptive effects against thermal stimuli is largely genetically independent of the mechanism by which morphine produces its antinociceptive effects against chemical stimuli, and (iv) inherent differences in sensitivity to painful stimuli may be responsible, in part, for individual differences in the potency of morphine's antinociceptive effects.[9]

Another paper looking into genetic influence on variability in human acute experimental pain sensitivity associated with gender, ethnicity, and psychological temperament demonstrated "that gender, ethnicity and temperament contribute to individual variation in thermal and cold pain sensitivity by interactions with TRPV1 and OPRD1 single nucleotide polymorphisms."[10]

Propranolol is a medication in the betablocker class usually used to treat high blood pressure and angina and to treat or prevent heart attacks. A study looked into possible effects of this medication for pain resulting from temporomandibular disorder (TMD) in a manner dependent on the subjects' *COMT* diplotype. (A *haplotype* is a group of genes inherited from a single parent. A *diplotype* is a pair of haplotypes from a given individual.) "A beneficial effect of propranolol on pain perception was noted in subjects not carrying this haplotype, a diminished benefit was observed in the heterozygotes, and no benefit was noted in the homozygotes."[11]

We physicians must be careful not to subscribe too closely to cultural stereotypes. Studies have found that some physicians prescribe medication in different doses depending on gender or even ethnicity.

David Weissman, Deb Gordon, and Shiva Bidar-Sielaff put their research on this subject into an article titled "Cultural Aspects of Pain Management." The article said, in part:

What is it about people that directs them to express their pain experience in different ways? Culture is the framework that directs human behavior in a given situation. The meaning and expression of pain are influenced by people's cultural background. Pain is not just a physiological response to tissue damage but also includes emotions and behavioral responses based on individuals' past experiences and perceptions of pain (e.g., when you were a child was your expressive behavior tolerated or were you expected to be stoic?).

Not everyone in every culture conforms to a set of expected behaviors or beliefs, so trying to categorize a person into a particular cultural stereotype (e.g., all North Dakota farmers are stoic) will lead to inaccuracies. On the other hand, knowledge of a patient's culture may help you better understand their behavior. [12]

A good example of how prejudice can worm itself into a physician's attitude was the frequent dismissal of complaints by women diagnosed with "chronic fatigue syndrome." Because females were believed to be prone to overstating physical ailments, this affliction was often marginalized—until it became known as fibromyalgia.

Again, according to Weismann, Gordon, and Bidar-Sielaff:

Even more important than understanding the culture of others is understanding how your own upbringing affects your attitude about pain. We are likely to believe that our reaction to pain is "normal" and that other reactions are "abnormal." Thus, a doctor or nurse from a stoic family may not know how to react to a patient who responds to pain by loud verbal complaints (or discount the pain because of the apparent mismatch between the injury and the verbal response). Even subtle cultural and individual differences, particularly in nonverbal, spoken, and written language, between health care providers and patients impact care. [13]

All of us, physicians and everyone else, must be careful of attaching our own values to other people. During the 2010 pro football playoffs, for instance, Chicago Bears quarterback Jay Cutler removed himself from a game with the Green Bay Packers with a knee injury that was later revealed to be painful but not serious. For the next several weeks, the sports Internet sites and talk radio stations were buzzing with a debate as to whether or not Cutler "wimped out." In other words, shouldn't a football player be more impervious to pain than the average person?

In the final analysis, we all belong to a cross-section of cultural groups—based on gender, ethnicity, religion, work, and so on. Beyond that, each human being on the planet is completely unique. No one else has the same exact set of life circumstances, genes, and experiences. No one else reacts to pain in quite the same way. No one else is programmed like you.

When he was running for office, former president Bill Clinton used to gaze out into his audiences and proclaim, "I feel your pain."

In reality, though, no one can truly do that. Not even your doctor.

7

THE STIGMA OF PAIN

Within American culture, two negative archetypes rise above (or, perhaps, sink below) all others—the drug addict and the laggard.

These individuals are reviled not only because of their perceived weakness but because they fail to contribute to society.

Given this, it's easy to see the problem faced by many with chronic pain. These archetypes are so prevalent that people on the borderline are often guilty until proven innocent. With someone suffering from fibromyalgia or chronic headaches or any of a dozen other unseen ailments, that proof can be difficult to produce.

For one thing, as I've already mentioned, the genesis of chronic pain can be far too complicated for the average person without medical training to absorb. Common knowledge tells us that people hurt because something very specific has hurt them. The idea that the brain and the network of nerves connected to it somehow can be mistaken seems suspicious.

Thus, those with chronic pain are struck by a double-edged sword—they are in pain and yet for some, those who matter to them may not believe that they are in pain. Sometimes, not even their physician believes them.

Take, for example, migraine headaches. As Laura Schocker wrote in the *Huffington Post*:

> Nearly 30 million Americans suffer from migraines, a condition characterized by crushing pain, frequently on one side of the head, that is often coupled with nausea and vomiting, sensitivity to light and

sound and sometimes even visual disturbances (known as auras). A single attack can take anywhere from six to 48 hours to run its course. This very specific type of headache often runs in families and is typically brought on by a variety of triggers, which may include physical or emotional stress, changes in sleep patterns, certain odors and bright lights, among many others.

But for a neurological condition as common as migraines, many people still doubt that it's a real condition. One recent study found that people with chronic migraines report feeling more rejected and ridiculed by friends, employers and even family members than patients with other types of neurological troubles, such as stroke, Parkinson's or Lou Gehrig's disease.[1]

Schocker quoted Jason Rosenburg, a professor of neurology at Johns Hopkins, who noted, "I see it from husbands and wives who roll their eyes at their spouse for saying they have headaches to employers not recognizing it as an illness."[2]

Kim Spangler of Niagara Falls, New York, has suffered from migraines for most of her adult life.

"Not only can't I do anything when I have them," she said, "but I often have to get away from everybody and go into a dark room. Sometimes, that makes people feel like you're pushing them away, so it's harder for them to sympathize."[3]

Again, Jason Rosenburg states: "It's not like the person is wheezing or there's a blood sugar test that can come high. Most diseases that people would see as 'legitimate' have a test or a scan."[4]

After all, *everyone* has headaches. *Everyone* has unexplained aches and pains, especially everyone over the age of thirty. For people who have not experienced a migraine, it leaves them wondering, what's the big deal?

As Rosenburg points out, there are two good reasons to develop better diagnostic recognition for many chronic pain ailments. Obviously, such tests would help with treatment, but a further advantage would be to help patients justify their ailments to others.

Diabetes might be one example. Often there are no physical symptoms to set a person with high blood sugar apart from anyone else. Yet when that person can say, "I checked my sugar and it was over 250," it makes the problem seem more real because there is a number attached. Similarly, a temperature of 104 means trouble almost universally.

Still, there is more to public skepticism of chronic pain than simply medical ignorance. As we addressed some of these cultural differences regarding pain in the previous chapter, people with these conditions often run afoul of that faint strain of Calvinism still present in America and other Western cultures.

This is a sticking point when it comes to pain-killing drugs, especially opioids. A Calvinist might be convinced that it's permissible to ingest these medications to reduce pain and get back to work, but the experience should never be enjoyable.

During the late 1960s and early 1970s, however, a cultural divide cracked open and spread between the so-called flower children and the previous generation. In the process, drug use became a major issue, especially when it was flaunted by the young. Along with long hair, loud music, and a propensity to vote for liberal politicians, recreational drug indulgence became either a badge of honor or a stain of dishonor, depending on the generational perspective.

Eventually, this led to the growing conviction that drug use had come to threaten the very fabric of society, with some chronic pain patients caught in the crossfire. We'll discuss that in detail later.

What this means for these patients (already suspect because of the vague nature of their illness) is that they are often seen not only as using their condition to avoid the responsibility of being productive but as a backdoor to pleasurable drugs.

However, this argument does not take into account all the reasons chronic pain sufferers abuse their medications. Some patients may overuse these drugs because the prescribed amount does not seem to be sufficient. Very few individuals will say, with honesty, that having to keep discomfort at bay with a steady parade of pills is an ideal existence.

As for the charge of laziness, most chronic pain sufferers would much rather be busy and productive than idle and stigmatized.

All of this is bad enough for a person with chronic back pain. What is even worse is when the medical establishment to which that patient goes seeking help is unsympathetic.

In 1998, a Fresno State University psychology professor named Marcia Bedard presented a paper at the annual meeting of the Society for Disability Studies titled "Bankruptcies of the Heart: Secondary Losses from Disabling Chronic Pain." In it, she directly confronted the idea that most individuals claiming chronic pain did so seeking idleness, sympathy, or drugs.

"For more than 30 years now," Bedard wrote, "the majority of psychologists have been shifting their emphasis toward treating chronic pain as a perceptual and psychological phenomenon rather than a true medical problem. One of the major theorists in this field was Wilmer Fordyce, who developed an influential social-learning model of chronic pain based on behaviorism about 20 years ago. Fordyce believed that pain is behavior designed to protect oneself or solicit aid and that pain increases, i.e., this behavior is strengthened, when followed by desirable consequences."[5]

According to Bedard, Fordyce listed the four most common "secondary gains" as "1. Attention and sympathy from family, friends and physicians; 2. Release from task responsibilities at home and at work; 3. Narcotic medications presumed to induce constant euphoria and 4. Monetary compensation which approximates actual wages."[6]

Bedard countered this with her own list of four "secondary losses": "1. Anger/trivialization/rejection by family, friends and physicians; 2. Complicated/frustrating tasks dealing with new bureaucracies; 3. Agonizing pain without medication; unpleasant side effects with medication and 4. Denial of disability benefits to which they are legally entitled."[7]

In her paper, Bedard made a telling argument that Fordyce's "gains" tended to be ephemeral, most often because of the longevity of chronic pain.

Sympathy, it seems, has a shelf life. Whether it is a spouse or a family physician, human beings are generally oriented toward solving problems. A husband or wife will gladly take greater responsibility for the children or the housework to help their loved one recover from an illness or injury but will understandably become frustrated and angry when that added burden drags on for months or years.

In fairness, that anger is most often directed not at the patient but at the circumstances. Nevertheless, it is the chronic pain sufferer who bears the brunt of it.

Nor, Bedard pointed out, are physicians immune to this withdrawal.

"Attention and sympathy from physicians," she said, "may be absent at the onset of chronic pain, but if not, it generally wanes as the patient fails to respond to one after another medical interventions, leaving most doctors feeling frustrated and helpless. Patients with incurable, irreversible and progressive conditions, such as degenerative disk and joint disease, may have a difficult time even finding a doctor who will take them as a patient. Consequently, many chronic pain patients are literally 'fired' by their treating physicians a year or so after numerous painful and invasive treatments have been tried and failed, and left on their own to try and find another doctor."[8]

Fortunately, in the fourteen years since Bedard delivered that paper, there has been some improvement, at least regarding physicians. Whereas the balance was once tipped heavily toward skeptics in the medical profession, it has gradually shifted more toward a level equilibrium. Even so, chronic pain is still not a major focus of medical school curriculums, and chronic pain patients are often not welcomed by general practitioners because they don't fit well into the logistics of today's overcrowded medical system.

On the plus side, it has become easier to find a specialist who will validate chronic pain symptoms, and the Internet is full of support groups for every imaginable condition. Yet exchanging sympathy in a chat room is not the same as receiving it at home.

Many chronic pain patients have to make a subconscious, and conscious, decision as to how much agony to "present" to the outside. This can lead to persistent, ongoing stress. Showing off too much for too long can risk losing the initial sympathy. Not expressing what they may be going through risks suffering in silence.

In her introduction to a paper titled "Stigma, Liminality and Chronic Pain," Jean Jackson of the Massachusetts Institute of Technology (MIT) pointed out:

> I argue here that certain features of chronic pain can result in sufferers being seen to transgress the categorical division between mind and body and to confound the codes of morality surrounding sickness and health. As a consequence, they threaten the normal routines of biomedical treatment and the expectations governing ordinary face-to-face interactions between individuals labeled "sick" and the rest of the social world.[9]

Essentially, the average person groups illness or injury into two categories: temporary or terminal. Most chronic pain disorders are neither. Even worse, it is often unclear whether the affliction is "fixable" or not.

In a small way, it was no doubt helpful when dancer, singer, and *American Idol* judge Paula Abdul told *People* magazine in 2005 that she was a long-time sufferer from reflex sympathetic dystrophy (RSD)/complex regional pain syndrome (CRPS), which she said stemmed from a teenaged cheerleading injury. In the course of her treatment, Abdul noted, she had taken OxyContin, Vicodin, Soma, and other opioid drugs.[10]

The issue of her RSD/CRPS surfaced when Abdul appeared confused on *American Idol*—a side effect not only of the disease but the medication employed to treat it—and a prairie fire of rumors leaped across entertainment TV and the Internet, speculating that she was either "on drugs" or an alcoholic.

For the most part, her explanation appeared to be accepted by Abdul's fans and the media and even led to a small and short flurry of RSD-related news articles. Moreover, in a culture where some diseases don't seem real until they are contracted by a celebrity (Rock Hudson and AIDS, Michael J. Fox and Parkinson's disease), perhaps all this gave the thousands of RSD sufferers who never appeared on camera permission to be who they are.[11]

None of these short-lived articles or network features, however, had the fierce power of Marcia Bedard's hardly noticed 1998 talk to a small group of people who probably agreed with her.

Speaking of the "secondary gain" theory, she said:

> This is, in my estimation, nothing short of institutional moral larceny: a victim-blaming ploy that serves primarily to justify the reprehensible actions of insurance companies, opposing attorneys, and many of the private, county, state and federal bureaucracies purporting to "assist" persons with disabilities. Secondary gain, or any other concept built on myths and stereotypes which contribute to ongoing discrimination against persons disabled by chronic pain needs to be exposed for what it is—unconscionable in a democratic society.
>
> What is desperately needed at this point . . . is a massive public education campaign regarding the enormous losses, tangible and intangible, that accompany disabling chronic pain.[12]

I can only hope that this book might be part of that solution.

8

SAD BUT TRUE—CHRONIC PAIN AND DEPRESSION

It is hopelessness, even more than pain that crushes the soul.

—William Styron

On any number of levels, chronic pain is depressing.

Although acute pain is often more hurtful and debilitating than its chronic counterpart, it usually comes with a shelf life that gives hope to those it afflicts. Here, a patient is told his or her pain will lessen in a week, a little more the following week, then continue to decrease until he or she is finally able to resume normal activities. That prospect makes the worst of the discomfort easier to bear because the patient sees light at the end of the tunnel.

For people with chronic pain, however, it is as if the end of the tunnel has been sealed up and bricked over. This 2011 excerpt from the blog of a fibromyalgia sufferer no doubt eloquently speaks for thousands of others:

> I honestly don't know how I've made it this far and I don't know how much longer I can do this. The pain gets worse every year and I've lost so much from it. I have very few friends. I almost never go anywhere. I spend significant amounts of time stuck in bed due to pain and not being able to walk. I'm just so tired of it and terrified of what my life will be like two years from now, or 5 or 10. The desire to just give up and disconnect from life completely (not suicide, but

unplugging my mind . . . catatonic) has been extremely tempting and strong these past couple weeks.

I've become something I fought against so long. I've become a burden to others.

I hate it. [1]

In dealing with chronic pain, a physician must always consider a patient's mental state as well as physical condition. The problem is, there is a tendency in the medical profession to regard depression as merely an appendage to pain. Fix the pain and the depression will vanish automatically. Sometimes that's true. But depression can also become a major obstacle thrown in the path of treatment options, and there are times when the two afflictions can embrace in a dark dance, spiraling downward.

I don't necessarily consider myself pro- or anti-medication when it comes to depression. I do believe, however, that it is first necessary to evaluate the patient and determine what might be done to draw them out and improve their mood, and lifestyle, without simply writing a prescription.

An important part of the equation is whether the depression is situational or clinical. Chronic pain not only hurts physically, but its impact ripples outward into all aspects of a person's life. Job performance is often affected, which may lead to unemployment. Activities that once relieved stress become difficult. Someone in serious chronic pain often becomes unable to contribute to housework or yardwork. Sexual activity may cease.

In other words, pain that refuses to go away can expand to fill up a patient's life, crowding out everything that once gave it vibrancy and meaning. No wonder that person becomes depressed—who wouldn't?

When I begin seeing a new patient, I always try to look at the things about them that may be relevant to the patient's management. This includes whether the patient has a strong, understanding support system in place or whether years of dealing with the patient's pain issues have worn away the patience of other family members. Has the patient maintained important friendships, or has he or she drifted away, with no one to talk to and lean on? In the case of the elderly, they may be living alone and may not have a structured support system or family around to help take care of them. Finding ways to climb out of isolation and build a support system has to be part of the initial conversation with those solitary sufferers.

More than anything, some people in chronic pain are looking for information and a context to understand their condition. It might be religious or spiritual. It might be hopeful, as in the promise of a new drug. It might even be a dogged determination not to let the pain win. Patients in the latter category may benefit just from knowing what is causing their suffering. They are then more amenable to modalities like psychological support and physical therapy. Even if the actual pain relief may not be considerable, these offer the powerful incentive of participation in their own treatment. They are doing something proactive rather than just sitting on their couches watching television and waiting for the next pill to kick in.

Others simply need to talk about their situation or solicit suggestions on ways to cope with it mentally. Every pain doctor must have a certain amount of counseling skill but should also be willing to trust the judgment of a professional psychiatrist or psychologist when things do not seem to be going right.

"I asked to go to counseling," said one of my patients, who was simultaneously grappling with fibromyalgia, arthritis, and lupus. "My family was supportive, but I just felt I needed a professional to get me through it. I was too depressed to get out of bed for a while, and my kids needed me."

She was one of the fortunate ones. As Kathleen Crowley put it in a 1996 article for the National Pain Outreach Association,

> The very nature of depression is at odds with the treatment of it. Severe depression can be defined in one word—hopelessness. A severely depressed person has no hope for the future and no memory of things ever having been any different. Swallowing a pill may be the only action a severely depressed individual is initially capable of.[2]

But according to a 2007 article in the *Psychological Bulletin*, there is also a flip side. "Some have suggested that chronic pain is a form of 'masked depression,' whereby patients use pain to express their depressed mood because they feel it is more acceptable to complain of pain than to acknowledge that one is depressed."[3]

Moreover, one popular counseling definition of depression is "anger turned inward," and the aforementioned article also notes: "Depression and anxiety have received the greatest amount of attention in chronic pain patients; however, anger has recently received considerable interest as a significant emotion."[4]

Chronic pain patients who become angry activate their fight or flight reflex, thus creating stress and thereby often aggravating their condition.

Then there is the second type of depression, generally described as *clinical*.

Clinical depression and chronic pain actually have a lot in common. Both are conditions that until recently were viewed with some skepticism, not only by the general public but by elements of the medical community. Even now, many people don't see depression as a disease but rather a reaction to outside circumstances. Viewed in this context, a person who falls prey to the blues is not sick but weak.

"How could he have killed himself?" we sometimes hear when someone resorts to this radical and thoroughly unwarranted course. "He had a good job, a loving family. He had everything to live for."

Yet if that person was also suffering from clinical depression, this would be like making the same statement about someone who died of cancer. Unlike situational depression, the clinical variety exists in a vacuum, impervious to any brightness from outside.

A Harvard University study in 2004 reported evidence that depression and chronic pain even appear to share a neurological link:

> The convergence of depression and pain is reflected in the circuitry of the nervous system. In the experience of pain, communication between body and brain goes both ways. Normally, the brain diverts signals of physical discomfort so we can concentrate on the external world. When this shutoff mechanism is impaired, physical sensations, including pain, are more likely to become the center of attention. Brain pathways that handle the reception of pain signals, including the seat of emotions in the limbic region, use some of the same neurotransmitters involved in the regulation of mood, especially serotonin and norepinephrine. When regulation fails, pain is intensified along with sadness, hopelessness and anxiety. And chronic pain, like chronic depression, can alter the functioning of the nervous system and perpetuate itself.[5]

According to Stephen Stanos, medical director of the Chicago-based Chronic Pain Care Center,

> Studies show that depressed patients are more likely to report a greater number and severity of physical symptoms. In addition, chronic pain and depression show a significant clinical overlap with stress-related pain disorders such as chronic low back pain, facial pain, irritable bowel syndrome, migraine, phantom limb pain and temporomandibular disorders.
>
> A biopsychosocial model of chronic pain incorporates the physical, cognitive, affective and behavioral components related to the ongoing pain experience.[6]

Yet while *biopsychosocial* sounds impressive on paper, the most effective treatment plan ever devised won't work if a patient is too depressed to follow it.

Our bodies have natural defenses against depression. Exercise lifts our moods by raising endorphin levels. Yet what if physical activity is too painful (or the patient too depressed) for it to be a practical alternative?

Similarly, depressed individuals need a caring support system to avoid plunging into a bottomless emotional pit. At the same time, dealing with a depressed person often offers little positive feedback or emotional reward for friends and family. Often, in time, it becomes easier just to assume that the individual doesn't want company.

That may, indeed, be the case. But obsession often piggybacks on isolation, and if someone with chronic pain has no distractions, the hurt takes on a life of its own. Eventually, it is all that person thinks about and focuses on.

I remember one night when I developed a severe, painful toothache that lasted for hours. None of the over-the-counter medications I had in the house worked, and I started calling doctor friends to see if I could get something prescribed late at night. I got into a lengthy conversation with one of them, and when I hung up the phone, I realized that the pain was gone.

Such is the power of distraction, part of which goes back to the "pain gate" theory of Ronald Melzack and Patrick Wall. Other impulses to the brain pass through the same entrance as the harbingers of pain, and if there is enough general traffic, the pain impulses might get shoved to the side.

There are really three possibilities why a person with chronic pain might also seem depressed:

1. The depression could, as previously mentioned, be nothing more than a normal human reaction to a sad situation. Such individuals often benefit from counseling and/or exercise, and both of those weapons should be given high priority.
2. Since it has been proven that antidepressants help moderate pain whether depression is present or not, it could be that the same physiological factors sometimes cause both. The pain and the depression might be the result of the same malfunction of the nervous system.
3. The patient was already depressed, either clinically or situationally, before the chronic pain began to manifest itself.

"When you turn up a rheostat to control your kitchen light," says Dr. Rollin Gallagher, former editor in chief of the National Pain Foundation's newsletter,

> the light gets brighter and brighter. Well, that's what happens with your pain level when stress, bad mood, sadness or depression occurs at the same time as pain. Thus, a low-level pain signal, say from a chronic back condition—a level that normally you might be able to cope with—all of a sudden starts bothering you much more because the pain signal is amplified.
>
> The strong relationship between mood and pain is established in the medical literature by the research and through patients' own experiences. When someone has chronic pain that impairs functioning, which it normally does, the rates of clinical depression are from 30% to 80%, depending on which groups of patients and which type of pain.[7]

Indeed, chronic pain—difficult as it is to deal with medically—is sometimes easier to fix than depression. The drug Cymbalta, for example, was originally launched with an ad campaign related to mood enhancement. But when it was discovered that it also worked on chronic pain, the television ads switched to that audience.

As a physician, it's easy to see how certain drugs attack the two conditions differently. A drug like Cymbalta will generally begin to work on chronic pain in several days. By contrast, it often takes weeks for patients to notice a positive change in their mood.

Some patients who come to me have already fallen into the trap of self-medicating their depression with alcohol or drugs. Others are taking as many as four or five different types of antidepressants simultaneously. Not only can this be counterproductive but it can be life threatening. That's why it's so important that each of the physicians treating a particular patient be on the same page.

Alcohol is also a culprit in many fatal drug overdoses. We tend to look at it as something separate from any medication we've been taking, so washing potent pills down with several drinks doesn't seem dangerous. The fact is, of course, that alcohol exacerbates and accelerates the serious effects of most drugs.

One of the many debates currently underway in the chronic pain field is whether to first treat the depression, then the pain, or the other way around. Or should they be treated simultaneously?

Fortunately, some antidepressants—like the aforementioned Cymbalta—have been found to ease chronic pain symptoms whether the patient is depressed or not.

"The painkilling mechanism of these drugs is still not fully understood," states a 2011 report from the Mayo Clinic. "Antidepressants may increase neurotransmitters in the spinal cord that reduce pain signals. But they don't work immediately. You may feel some relief from an anti-depressant after a week or so, but maximum relief may take several weeks. Pain relief from antidepressants generally is moderate."[8] A British study at Oxford University reported:

> Antidepressants have two roles in managing chronic pain. The primary role is when pain relief with conventional analgesics (from aspirin or paracetamol through to morphine) is inadequate or when pain relief is combined with intolerable or unmanageable adverse effects. The failure of conventional analgesics should justify a therapeutic trial of antidepressants, particularly if the pain is neuropathic.[9]

My focus has always been on function. In prescribing medication, the trick is to provide enough of a dose to minimize the pain and allow the patient to resume something close to a normal life but not so much that he or she feels heavily drugged. The latter state quickly becomes counterproductive because it prevents the patient from moving forward in recovery.

Thus, when a new patient seems depressed, I first consider alternatives to mood-enhancing drugs that might be latched onto as life rafts in a sea of pain. Sometimes patients come in feeling very isolated and hopeless, either from lack of a support system at home or frustrated that nothing seems to be helping. Just listening to them can often give them the sense that there is someone on their side. A simple question like asking them to describe their pain and then patiently listening to them can be therapeutic.

In other cases, it becomes obvious that a patient needs counseling beyond what I am trained to deliver. Pain management is usually multidisciplinary, and psychiatric treatment often finds its way into the mix.

In recent years, there has been more of an emphasis on training doctors in the "people" aspect of their job. As difficult as it can be, it is always best to tread a fine line between realistic information and hope. A depressed person in chronic pain doesn't need to have all possibility of healing snatched away, although a tactfully presented worst-case scenario might be just the thing to inspire him or her to take treatment suggestions more seriously.

This is why psychiatry is one of the four disciplines in which physicians can train before they go for advanced training in pain management. The other three are anesthesiology, neurology, and physical medicine and rehabilitation or physiatry. An effective chronic pain specialist learns to recognize which patients need gentle encouragement and which require more sustained and continued efforts.

Certainly, chronic pain sufferers can be difficult to work with, especially when their affliction is combined with depression. These are the patients who sadly reply, in a barely audible voice, "I've tried that" or "That would never work" to every suggestion. If you are the latest in a series of medical options and all the others have failed, they may enter your office in a negative, even combative, frame of mind.

Being human, we will all experience self-pity at one time or another. Most of us, however, don't wallow in it. In part, because our situation invariably changes. With chronic pain sufferers, a change in their situation seems impossible. Thus, self-pity can become a way of life and a contributing factor to a downward pain-depression spiral.

Exact relation between depression and chronic pain has been the subject of much speculation and research. Does one lead to the other, and how? Are both a by-product of changes in the function, structure, or compounds in and around the brain tissue? Physicians have to decide on treatment priorities when both conditions coexist. Fortunately, there are many common remedies.

Still, crossing that bridge on a patient-to-patient basis isn't always easy. Despite the common image of chronic pain sufferers as craving and demanding stronger and stronger mind-altering drugs, many actually resist antidepressants at first. Depressed people often don't see themselves as depressed. When suggesting that they may benefit from antidepressants, responses are usually, "I'd be fine if only my [back, head, knee] would stop hurting."

I always smile when I remember one such patient of mine who was suffering with depression and chronic neuropathy from diabetes for many years. I decided to start her on duloxetine because this medication works on both.

At her next follow-up, she had half the pain and a major improvement in mood. She reported that she had been able to indulge in interactions and activities that she could not do in years.

9

OBESITY AND CHRONIC PAIN

On the face of it, one might wonder why there is a chapter on obesity in a book about chronic pain. In the next few pages, we will try to discuss the rationale.

A pleasant, fiftyish, morbidly obese female patient made an appointment recently to see me in my office. She had been to the pain center at the university hospital in our town with chronic pain from severe osteoarthritis of her knees and also pain in her back. She was almost in tears because, according to her, she was told by the resident physician that she was "too fat" and he could not do anything for her unless "she lost weight." This was not the first time I was faced with a situation like this. Though I, too, realized that many of her health issues, including chronic pain, were possibly linked to her overweight status, I had to tread respectfully and present my workup and recommendations honestly, without offending her further.

In my practice, I often deal with difficult situations like this. I have to focus on the complex intricacies of chronic pain while taking into account other conditions, such as obesity and other comorbid conditions. I have to think about how corelated these conditions are and how best to devise a mutually agreed upon management plan.

A study based on the electronic health records of the Veterans Health Administration concludes that obesity is significantly and consistently associated with persistent pain complaints.[1] Another major multistate study reveals an incremental relationship between obesity and pain; pain complaints became more prevalent as BMI status rose. The likelihood of morbidly obese people having a pain complaint was four times higher than those who were not obese.[2] There is a complex web of interactions between obesity, chronic pain, and other comorbid conditions that has been well researched and documented.

Obesity is a condition of abnormal or excessive fat accumulation in adipose tissue. It is usually defined by using weight and height to calculate a person's body mass index (BMI) and measured in kilograms per square meter (kg/m^2). Normal weight status ranges from 18.5 to 24.9, and overweight status ranges from 25 to 29.9. A BMI that is greater than 30 is considered obese. The obese category is further subdivided into class I (30–34.9), class II (35–39.9), and class III ($\geq$40). A BMI that is greater than 40 is considered "morbid" obesity.

According to the recent estimates by the World Health Organization (WHO), 39 percent and 13 percent of adult populations worldwide were overweight and obese in 2014, respectively.[3] In the United States, the rate of obesity seems to far exceed the world average.

A recent large-scale study with over nine thousand participants found that 69 percent of the participating adults were either overweight or obese and 35 percent were in the obese category.[4] Further, this study explains:

> Obesity and chronic pain both present serious public health concerns. The two conditions appear to co-occur frequently and likely have reciprocally negative impact on one another. Although as clinical syndromes, pain and obesity are significantly associated with each other, research evaluating the relationship between obesity and pain sensitivity has yielded conflicting results. This suggests that the relationship between obesity and pain is not a direct one but is mediated by various factors. Such factors include biomechanical/structural changes associated with obesity, inflammatory mediators, mood disturbance, poor sleep, and lifestyle issues. In particular, research on potential chemical mediators linking obesity with pain is rapidly growing. Those interested in further discussion on this topic may be interested in excellent reviews recently published. These papers also address various potential mediators relevant to specific pain diagnoses as well. It is, however, important to note that all of these mediating factors are implicated in the obesity-pain link in diverse ways across patients; that is, the relevance of these factors may vary greatly from a person to person. Multivariate assessment of patients and consolidation of all relevant biopsychosocial information are es-

sential in understanding how obesity and chronic pain are inter-twined in each patient. In general, losing weight, either via surgical intervention or via behavioral intervention (i.e., diet and exercise), appears to be beneficial for pain and associated QOL. A challenge however seems to be the long-term maintenance of benefit. All treatments require patients to internalize adaptive eating habits and staying active, which are not easy tasks even for healthy people. Further research is needed to develop posttreatment strategies to help patients maintain weight loss.[5]

In the majority of cases, obesity is the by-product of input and output. How much food is consumed and how much is burned by activity. I remember reading about a multidecade, multimillion-dollar government study to look at the effects of the diets and nutritional programs in the general population. The conclusion, in essence, was watch what (or, actually, how much) you eat.

There are no magic potions that will miraculously melt away those excess pounds.

In an article on the dietary approach to treatment of obesity, Angela Makris and Gary Foster report,

Popular dietary approaches for weight loss have generated wide-spread interest and considerable debate. While energy balance remains the cornerstone of weight control (i.e., calories still count), new diets and books promising weight loss by limiting certain foods or macronutrients rather than energy are constantly emerging and hitting the best seller list. Although their names and approaches may change over time, their basic premise has not. They market "success" as a large weight loss over a short period with little effort. Given the allure of a quick fix, overweight and obese individuals are often in search of the next "best" diet. The public's willingness to try diverse and, in some cases, poorly researched dietary approaches underscores their long-standing struggle to control their weight and the need for more effective strategies to help create an energy deficit. In order to develop more effective strategies, it is important to understand the efficacy, health effects, and long-term sustainability of current dietary approaches to weight control.

Various dietary strategies can effectively reduce weight, as shown by this review. Those that are coupled with behavior therapy and ongoing support tend to produce longer lasting effects. Improvements in health parameters are observed with each dietary strategy. Improvements in diabetes and CVD (cerebrovascular disease) risk factors have been observed with diets ranging from 10% fat to 45% fat. HP diets seem to be particularly effective in reducing fat mass and TAG, especially in individuals with dyslipidemia and who are at risk for type 2 diabetes. Likewise, LC diets have been shown to be effective in decreasing TAG (triglycerides) and VLDL (very-low-density lipoproteins) and increasing HDL (high density lipoprotein). Although low GI diets do not seem to be superior to any other diet for weight loss, there is evidence to suggest that they may provide some metabolic benefit for those with type 2 diabetes.

Clearly, all of these diets have benefits but they can only be realized when they are followed. A common theme across studies is poor long-term adherence and weight regain. Dansinger et al. found a strong association between diet adherence and clinically significant weight loss, suggesting that "sustained adherence to a diet" rather than "following a certain type of diet" is the key to successful weight management.[6]

Some patients with chronic pain may not be morbidly obese but may fit into the category of metabolic syndrome, a lesser-known condition that has been the focus of the medical community recently. It is not a single disease but a combination of factors that lead to increased risks of diabetes, stroke, and cardiovascular disease. These factors include excess fat around the waist along with high cholesterol, triglycerides, blood sugar, and blood pressure levels. The risk factors include obesity, family history, and being of the African American race.

That brings us to the possibility of chemical changes that predispose, and maintain, chronic pain status. A recent study concluded that women with chronic pain from fibromyalgia are at an increased risk for metabolic syndrome, which may be associated with relatively elevated norepinephrine (NE) levels in conjunction with relatively reduced epinephrine and cortisol secretion.[7]

The aptly named website, the State of Obesity, which specifically studies, monitors, and advises on the issues related to obesity, illustrates the challenge clearly:[8]

1. "Obesity is a financial issue. The obesity crisis costs our nation more than $150 billion in healthcare costs annually and billions of dollars more in lost productivity."

2. "Obesity is a national security issue. The obesity crisis also impacts our nation's military readiness. Being overweight or obese is the leading cause of medical disqualifications, with nearly one-quarter of service applicants rejected for exceeding the weight or body fat standards."

3. "Obesity is a community safety issue. With millions of obese and overweight Americans serving as first responders, firefighters, police officers and in other essential community service and protection roles, public safety is at risk."

4. "Obesity is a child development and academic achievement issue. Obesity prevention is an investment in our children's ability to learn and grow."

5. "Obesity is an equity issue. Obesity disproportionately affects low-income and rural communities as well as certain racial and ethnic groups, including Blacks."

6. "Obesity is a top national priority. Americans (registered voters) rated obesity as the top health concern in the country in a recent public opinion survey conducted by the Greenberg, Quinlan, Rosner Research and Bellweather Research groups."

Federal, state and local agencies play a key role in creating and supporting policies that benefit millions of families and neighborhoods across America. Experts at the Centers for Disease Control and Prevention (CDC), National Institutes of Health (NIH), U.S. Department of Agriculture (USDA), U.S. Department of Education, the Administration for Children and Families (ACF), Food and Drug Administration (FDA), academic research centers and state and local public health agencies across the country have researched and developed top strategies for preventing and addressing obesity among children and adults. These include improving nutrition standards for the foods and beverages offered through the Child and Adult Care Food Program (CACFP) and in schools nationwide. These agencies also provide the evidence base and technical assistance for every school district in the country to develop effective, strategic, local wellness plans to identify "hot spots" where the problems are the most severe, the needs are the greatest and where promising efforts can be most effective. Communities, schools and families around the country rely on the expert technical assistance, guidance, toolkits and evaluations demonstrating effective efforts that can make a difference to improve health. These efforts allow communities to learn from the best evidence and programs, so they can build on them for the benefit of their own communities.

The individual decisions people make about eating and activity are not made in a vacuum. Where families live, learn, work and play all have a major impact on the choices they are able to make. Healthy foods are often more expensive and less available in some neighborhoods, and finding safe, accessible places and having time to be active can be challenging for many.

For instance, most children spend significant periods of time in child-care and schools where food options may be beyond the control of their parents.[9]

Having discussed the general implications and toll taken on society by obesity, let us circle back and look at the factors related not only to myofascial pain but also to neuropathic pain.

In 2015, Jun Hozumi and colleagues[10] presented a paper on the "Relationship between Neuropathic Pain and Obesity." In an article on Pain Research and Management, they conclude:

> Pain can be caused by a variety of physical and/or psychological factors, which are categorized as nociceptive, neuropathic, or a combination of both. Nociceptive pain is caused by tissue damage including musculoskeletal degeneration, vascular disease, and surgical wounds, as well as from injury to organs such as that due to cancer. The pathophysiological mechanism of nociceptive pain is the activation of the nociceptors located on the peripheral nerve endings, widely distributed in the peripheral tissue. The inflammatory molecules (e.g., bradykinin, prostaglandins, and serotonin) directly stimulate the nociceptors and cause inflammatory pain. Therefore, inflammatory pain is a form of nociceptive pain. A well-known explanatory theory of migraine is the trigeminovascular theory. Trigeminal activation causes the release of brain chemicals called neuropeptides (e.g., substance P, serotonin, and calcitonin gene-related peptide) and induces the dilation of the dural blood vessels on the brain surface, which results in local inflammation and pain. One of the pathophysiological mechanisms underlying migraine would be also known to be nociceptive/inflammatory pain. Considering these previous findings, obesity seems to aggravate nociceptive pain.
>
> The alternative pain mechanism is neuropathic. Neuropathic pain is defined as the pain caused by a lesion or a disease of the somatosensory nervous system and is not a diagnosis but a clinical

description. To our knowledge, unlike nociceptive pain, the relationship of neuropathic pain with obesity is not clear. Obesity certainly
affects some neural conditions, such as depression and cognitive dysfunction. Regarding the peripheral nervous system, electrophysiolog-
ical examinations demonstrated that the motor and sensory action
potentials are significantly impaired in obese subjects, and obesity
has been shown to elevate experimental heat pain threshold."[11]

Putting aside the debate on whether obesity leads to chronic pain or
the other way around, we now know that there are proven and well-
defined links between the two.

As a nation, we are facing the double whammy of morbid obesity
and chronic pain. As a pain physician, I am more than eager to face this
challenge head on and do my part to help fight it.

10

FINDING THE RIGHT SPECIALIST

Patient: "Doctor, it hurts when I do this."
Doctor: "Then don't do that."

—Henny Youngman, comedy routine

Pain is all around us. Pain specialists are not.

There are a number of explanations for this. Pain management is a relatively new specialty, one not offered by all of the traditional medical schools. It requires a different type of commitment that doesn't always mesh with the traditional role of a physician. This is further complicated with the stringent legal and administrative oversight under which the pain physicians, unlike any other specialty, have to operate. In addition, the recent medical graduates tend to go for specialties that offer a more relaxed lifestyle.

After training, some pain physicians are able to start their own practices. This solo status, of course, also has its downside. Doctors who work in conjunction with other doctors get more time off and can accept more patients. Lone chronic pain physicians quickly discover that the in-depth and time-consuming personal interaction demanded by our specialty can very quickly lead to a standing-room-only waiting room if the physician is not judicious in scheduling.

Although I always knew that a high percentage of Americans suffered from chronic pain and needed care, it didn't become real to me until I saw the number of patients coming through my office door. In my part of Virginia, some patients come to me from a more than fifty-mile radius. The fact that some of the other pain practices in the region have stopped accepting Medicaid and other low-paying insurance sends more patients to those who do.

John Loeser, a professor of neurology and anesthesiology at the University of Washington and one of the pioneers in the chronic pain field, sees many large hospitals more as part of the problem than as contributors to the solution.

"For large American hospitals, especially those associated with a medical school," he writes, "revenue generation is the major determinant of what services the institution will offer. MPC (multi-disciplinary pain clinics) is not seen as a value compared to cosmetic surgery."[1]

Beyond that, he adds, "payment to providers is skewed in favor of procedures and surgeries, putting great economic pressures on those who provide a personal service without a procedural intervention."[2]

All these are factors calculated to entice medical school graduates into more lucrative and less complicated areas of medical care. So, as Dr. Henry Adams points out on his website, ChronicPainDoctor.net, "We have more people now needing more and more varied health care due to the economics, demographic and lifestyle patterns molded by this nation than ever before. We also have less people than ever before, proportionately, who are able to competently care for those who need it."[3]

In this case, supply and demand is compromised. Chronic pain is a big business in terms of patients, and demand keeps going up. But instead of flocking to fill this demand, some of the nation's doctors are running away from it.

For doctors, like lawyers, police investigators, plumbers, and auto mechanics, are focused on solutions. As a general rule, we don't like uncertainty, and we try to avoid loose ends.

Most of the patients I see are passed along by others in my profession, because whatever afflicts them defies a definitive "fix." Conditions such as reflex sympathetic dystrophy (RSD) or fibromyalgia can resist detection by even the most sophisticated medical gadgetry.

All too often it comes down to this: The patient is in pain because he says he is. It can't be proven or disproven.

Pain specialists often find themselves summoned to courtrooms for this very reason. Whether a patient is incapacitated by chronic pain or motivated by fraud can be an insurance or workman's compensation issue representing hundreds of thousands of dollars.

Yet some types of chronic pain, like RSD or phantom limb pain, are intrinsically illogical and all but impossible to explain to a jury. Our bodies tell us we are in pain, even when there is no concrete evidence of it. In worst-case scenarios, the attending physician winds up throwing darts at an ever-revolving board, hoping to hit the right target by chance.

Such cases are particularly difficult for harassed primary care physicians with full waiting rooms. The typical fifteen-minute window for one-on-one consultation is almost always inadequate to fully digest the convoluted turns and dead ends experienced by someone with an undiagnosed hurt. Meanwhile, back among the filing cabinets and computers, insurance issues arise that may discourage the doctor from running certain tests or trying newer medications on the basis of unverifiable information.

In short, mysterious and relentless pain can very quickly poison a doctor-patient relationship. Society has created an unrealistic image of the healing profession, for which we physicians are partly to blame. The suffering individuals typically walk into a medical facility or doctor's office with the confident expectation that they will be healed.

That expectation grows even stronger when the doctor involved is a specialist. The patient wants to hear "Ah, I see the problem," not "Let's try this and see if it works."

A person in chronic pain is often tired, frustrated, and filled with unfocused anger. That anger very quickly shifts to the attending physician if good things don't happen quickly.

I remember prescribing a pain medication for a young woman with fibromyalgia and explaining to her that this was only a test to see if the drug would help. If it didn't help, I told her, it might be necessary to change the dosage or try another remedy. For this, I needed her objective feedback after a few days.

The next day she called my office and said, "That didn't help a bit. I'm going to find a new doctor." You sometimes want to bang your head against a wall.

Doctors can't control everything—especially the ebb and flow of a disease. In a report for the International Research Foundation for RSD/CRPS, Dr. Anthony Kirkpatrick wrote:

The natural history of a disease can be highly variable. A headache comes and goes, as does a backache. Similarly, the symptoms of RSD can come and go, especially in children. One of the things that seems predictable is when there is an acute exacerbation of a disease (whether it be a headache, low back pain or RSD), there is a tendency for the doctor to treat the disease at that point in time. But this is when the symptoms of a disease might decrease without treatment. Therefore, when the symptoms of a disease fluctuate, the doctor may take undue credit for the improvement.

Similarly, symptoms may worsen once treatment has begun. Even with an effective treatment, the doctor may be blamed unfairly for a bad outcome. [4]

Even drugs that do work shouldn't be the final answer unless the condition is terminal or obviously unfixable. When you have a patient who only wants to feel better and a doctor who only wants that patient to go away satisfied, the groundwork is laid for a sort of conspiracy against the body—dulling or overwhelming the pain so it doesn't hurt anymore without really unmasking what's behind the hurt.

Why is that bad? Because situations like this may lead to escalating dosages of medications and possibly to addiction. Because over time the patient may develop a tolerance to that medication. Because it isn't really responsible medicine.

In my practice, I often find that I have to tell patients what they don't want to hear. In some cases, it's that they need to get off the couch and into an exercise program, even though it might be uncomfortable at first. Other times, I need to remind them that a drug-induced haze isn't where they want to take up permanent residence.

Writing for the National Pain Foundation and advocating for primary care physicians (the first line of defense, along with emergency room staff, against chronic pain), Dr. Bill McCarberg put it this way:

We can lament the deplorable state of medicine today and get angry at our health insurance or managed care organization, but the reality is that you have a medical problem causing pain. Your primary care provider has not chosen to limit your access to tests or drugs, but he or she may deny access because of insurance issues. There is a place for complaining and standing up for your right to quality medical care, but being angry with your doctor will not get you the results you want. It may get you the requested MRI, but it leaves you with an adversarial relationship with one of the best advocates for your case—the primary care provider.[5]

Without question, chronic pain patients need advocates. That all-too-obvious chip on their shoulder may have been placed there by employers, relatives, friends, or others in their lives who imply very strongly that their pain is "all in your head."

If you have a good relationship with your primary care physician, however, there are ways in which you can make it easier for him or her to work with you.

For starters, try writing down some of your history with this pain— what medications you've tried, whether or not the discomfort fluctuates, its apparent place of origin, and so on. Then drop this document off at your doctor's office so that he or she can peruse it at a convenient time. A "pain diary" over the previous month or so is also a good idea.

Should you decide to move beyond your initial medical contact to other doctors or specialists, it does you no good to sever the paper trail. Even if you disagree with an earlier diagnosis or recommended medications, make sure to inform your new doctor of any conducted tests that might still be relevant. There is no need for redundancy that might put you in expensive conflict with your insurance provider.

Indeed, my experience has been that primary care physicians are generally more than happy to refer their chronic pain patients to me or some other pain specialist.

Part of this is because of all the factors listed above. Chronic pain cases generally eat up a disproportionate amount of a general practitioner's time, not to mention the stress of dealing with prickly patients or a condition that can't be cured, alleviated, or sometimes even identified.

In other cases, primary care physicians are scared. The American opioid crisis and drug overdose is rightfully on everyone's mind, placing physicians under unprecedented scrutiny. With a stroke of a pen on a small piece of paper, a doctor can unwittingly cross the legal line between pain healer and drug dealer.

Given this, a lot of doctors would prefer that someone else take that risk. Dashing out a prescription for an aspirin derivative is one thing; opening a pathway to OxyContin or methadone quite another.

The twenty-first century has ushered in a new breed of patient, with mixed results for doctors.

We have moved away from the days of 1960s TV shows like *Marcus Welby, MD* and *Ben Casey*, where doctors not only fixed their patients' physical problems but their dysfunctional lives, thanks to long consultations over coffee. These sages in white lab coats were brimming with knowledge, imminently patient, and as wise as Yoda.

Today, in place of saintly archetypes, the prime-time medical scene features cynical, wisecracking physicians like the titular character on *House* and the randy crew on *Grey's Anatomy*, where patients seem to take a backseat to other intrahospital activities.

By and large, however, the doctor remains an object of respect—an authority figure to his or her patients. The physician, after all, is the keeper of the flame of knowledge.

But there is an emerging threat to this exalted status: the Internet.

The Internet now has doctors on it, even specialists. You can type in questions and get answers. However, they will, by necessity, be general answers that won't get the online doctor sued. Thus, instead of passively accepting what they're told by a doctor in his or her office, many people now plunge into researching their particular condition online, clicking on everything from reputable doctor-fed sites to patient-run chat rooms.

If this is done with a certain amount of perspective, it can prove helpful. Indeed, the consensus online may echo what a patient's doctor is telling him or her. Since the average busy general practitioner doesn't have time to track the latest news on every ailment known to man, some of this information might even be useful.

The problem comes when the seeker is bombarded with contradictory or, in some cases, blatantly inaccurate information. Posters on a chat room, most of whom have little or no medical knowledge, might respond to a question with everything from "I wouldn't worry about it" to "That's exactly what killed my uncle."

Dr. B. Eliot Cole, executive director of the American Society of Pain Educators, argues that the idea is not to try to one-up the doctor in his or her own field but rather to make sure the patient is given due respect:

> I hope patients will just get the point. You don't have to hurt. People suffer a lot more than they need to. And if they took a bit of action and became a so-called bad patient, became a little disruptive, said, "You know, this isn't *your* arm that hurts, it's *my arm*, and I want referral now, not in six months," things would be better.[6]

A productive doctor-patient relationship is a two-way street because both participants have information the other needs. Chances are the doctor knows a lot more about sickness and injury and treatment than you—it is, after all, his or her profession. Then again, the one subject on which nearly every human being is an expert is his or her own body. You know better than anyone else whether something hurts and where and when.

Thus, as they work together to turn a life of pain into something more manageable, both doctor and patient must bring certain things to the partnership.

Patients have the right to a doctor who listens to them and trusts them. Doctors need the patient to follow through on his or her recommendations and prescriptions.

So why choose a pain specialist over a general practitioner?

A well-trained and experienced pain specialist is better suited to deal with most cases of chronic pain. First and foremost, this was the focus of the specialist's training, which probably included anesthesiology, neurology, physical medicine, and psychiatry. This knowledge helps the pain specialist simultaneously focus on a multitude of factors that are involved in chronic pain. Second, only the pain specialist is able to offer, and perform, advanced interventional procedures, including nerve block, ablations, and neuromodulation techniques with peripheral and spinal cord stimulators. These minimally invasive interventional approaches are an essential part of most pain management protocols and afford optimum benefits when employed early in the course of disease.

It pains me to see some patients with conditions like reflex sympathetic dystrophy (RSD)/complex regional pain syndrome (CRPS) who are referred much later, when they have already developed muscle and bone loss, frequently resulting in loss of limb function. Chances are that they would have responded much better to an early instituted combination of aggressive physical therapy and nerve blocks.

Of course, not all chronic pain patients are candidate for interventional procedures, but many are. These interventions, employed early, offer significant advantages:

- Targeted relief of symptoms, allowing early rehabilitation
- Minimization of the risks of polypharmacy
- Longer lasting—no daily pills
- Safe in trained hands
- Better compliance
- Better in working adults and elderly
- Rare contraindications

Chuck Weber, spokesman for the American Pain Society, explains, "Pain is physical, it's emotional, it's psychological, it's social, it's economic."[7]

Thus, a multifaceted problem requires a multifaceted approach. In most cases, this means some medications, procedures, and physical therapy. Some patients benefit from referrals for psychological and psychiatric help.

In large cities, these specialists are sometimes grouped together in a clinic or multiple-practice setting. In other cases, they may be a single-specialty group practice. Wherever you live, an Internet search for "pain specialists" will summon forth a list of qualified, board-certified pain physicians, which is what you should be looking for. The American Board of Anesthesiology and other boards usually have a searchable, online list of professionals.

My focus, more than anything else, is restoring as much function as possible to the patient. This means, ideally, being able to work and participate in everyday activities. In many cases, medications should be a small, preferably temporary, recourse until more long-term approaches and interventions take effect.

What I like about specializing in chronic pain is that it is a dynamic, ever-changing field. Some branches of medicine seem to have reached a comfortable dead end, nudged forward only slightly by an occasional advancement in medication or intervention. Chronic pain research is still in its youth—remember, fibromyalgia wasn't recognized as a legitimate condition until the 1980s.

I've also found my relationship with many patients to be immensely gratifying. If someone goes to see a family doctor with a case of the flu, it's more than expected that the physician will make it better. People often come to me after trying many solutions, and several doctors, and they are running low on hope. They see no end to their torment. If I can show them even a glimpse of a resolution, they are often extremely grateful.

And so am I.

11

SEARCHING FOR THE CAUSE OF PAIN

Based on the current popularity of the rapidly multiplying *CSI*-type television programs, a lot of people seem to love a good mystery. So do I.

Indeed, that is one of the things that keeps me engaged in my job. Even better, unlike the on-screen crime scene investigators, who tend to look more like models than technicians, my mysteries involve real and living people.

Unfortunately, I get the feeling that many physicians have lost that sense of playing sleuth. In overworked, overbooked offices, "face time" is often kept to a minimum and patients are sent on their way clutching a prescription or two. The hope is that the medication will work and the mystery will resolve itself without the need for further investigation.

My patients, by contrast, have been down that road. They have been seen by general practitioners, tried more than one drug, and been referred to me because their chronic pain has not responded to standard intervention.

The one thing all of these poor souls have in common is that they hurt. But why? And what can I do about it?

First, I ask all my patients to fill out a rather lengthy questionnaire in advance of their initial visit. This may tell me what started the pain, what sort of pain they have been experiencing, where it seems to be located, how long it has lasted, and perhaps something about its severity and cycles. I also want to know their treatment history.

Meanwhile, I also try to get as much information as possible from the referring physician. Some patients have been passed along to me rather quickly after it became obvious that the previous doctor was faced with something beyond his or her experience. Others, in their frustration, have tried several different physicians and have already accumulated a rather lengthy medical dossier.

Either way, my intent is to hit the ground running as a health provider. With the patient's background in hand, I can spend more time asking detailed questions about what might be hurting him or her.

At the same time, I try to minimize the expense to the patient by not duplicating tests that have already been done. Most of the referring physicians with whom I work are professional and thorough, and chances are they have already done MRI and CT scans and blood work. If so, there is no reason to go back over that road, because nothing will have changed in such a short time.

What I hope will emerge from the initial consultation are some basic starting points:

1. Is the patient in extreme pain, or is this more of an annoyance?
2. How long has the pain been present? If it seems serious, and considerable time has elapsed, that obviously effects how quickly treatment is initiated.
3. Could the pain be coming from a previous injury?
4. To what extent has function been affected? Is the patient now out of work? Using a walker or a wheelchair?
5. How does the current physical situation compare with the patient's earlier ability to function?
6. How is the patient's mental state? Does the patient seem depressed? If so, I will often refer him or her to a counselor or psychiatrist. The better the patient's emotional attitude, the more of a coplayer the patient is likely to be in his or her own treatment.
7. What sort of support system surrounds this person? Is the patient elderly and alone or blessed with a helping family?

What a pain physician must avoid, at all costs, is tunnel vision. Some of the conditions that provoke chronic pain mimic other conditions. Still others offer no tangible symptoms at all. Patience is paramount here, because it might take several appointments before a likely cause is rooted out.

The most common causes of chronic pain will be discussed in chapter 13—including back and spinal injuries, arthritis, migraine and other types of headaches, multiple sclerosis, fibromyalgia, RSD/CRPS, post-shingles syndrome and neuropathy.

Like those TV detectives, pain doctors are often forced to operate by eliminating suspects, one by one. Sometimes the culprit can be the most obvious, but physicians should also be prepared to be surprised.

A 2011 article from the Cleveland Clinic describes how complex this procedure can be:

> The traditional tests used to diagnose painful conditions include X-rays, magnetic resonance imaging (MRI), electromyography (EMG), and nerve conduction studies. However, tests that are often performed in pain management centers are directed toward eliminating or reducing pain as an endpoint.
>
> For example, while EMG and nerve conduction studies might tell health care providers what is wrong with a particular nerve or nerves, blocking these structures with a local anesthetic can help the health care provider distinguish between pain that might be arising within a nerve or nerves, or from the structures that they serve. Such tests might involve the sequential blocking of a peripheral nerve, the nerve root from which it arises, or a structure within the spinal canal, for example.
>
> Often, because there is an interplay between different types of nerves—such as sympathetic, motor, and sensory fibers—some of the injection techniques are used to distinguish their respective roles in the production of pain by having as an endpoint a change in function or pain. For example, blocking the ability of a particular muscle or joint to move.
>
> Certain conditions, such as reflex sympathetic dystrophy—which is now known as complex regional pain syndrome (CRPS)—are associated with a disturbance of the circulation to the skin and deeper structures. Diagnostic tests can be done to observe the change in temperature when sympathetic nerves, which control this circulation, are blocked.
>
> In this instance, thermography is used to measure these temperature changes dynamically and can be a great help in establishing a diagnosis. Similarly, as anybody who has backaches knows, chronic

pain symptoms might continue after otherwise satisfactory surgery when a mechanical defect is repaired. Pain arising from structures around the spine has multiple causes, often without satisfactory evidence by the different imaging techniques. A common pain (backache) that remains after surgery can be identified by muscle dysfunction and can be confirmed by the use of trigger point injections, which can also facilitate its treatment.

The sympathetic nervous system has been shown to participate in many pain conditions, not infrequently after a pre-existing injury. Unless this is recognized through appropriate diagnostic testing, this type of pain will remain, no matter how many analgesics (pain killers) and other treatments are used.[1]

Quite naturally, some patients who are in severe pain arrive in my office wanting immediate and total relief. This presents a dilemma for the physician. Even if I were to take away all the pain—for example, with a pain pill—that would make it even more difficult to find the source. Sometimes it's necessary to strike a balance between making the patient more comfortable and temporarily leaving enough of the pain to announce its presence and location.

There is also a necessary element of experimentation: trying a low dose of a pain medicine to see how much it helps, blocking a nerve that appears to be the seat of the problem while realizing that the offending nerve may actually be located somewhere else. My sense of the medical profession is that a doctor shouldn't be afraid to be wrong if a procedure is done in good faith and as long as the guesswork is not endangering the patient—especially if the alternative is doing nothing.

It is important, though, to make sure the patient is informed and consulted every step of the way. Even if the source of someone's chronic pain can be identified, what approaches to use and what restorative procedure to undertake may sometimes depend on the individual's physical and emotional state.

Like every other physician, I gain considerable satisfaction from the "Ah ha!" moments when an initial hunch is validated. But when all the diagnostic tricks in my bag fail, I have learned to shift the emphasis from cure to management.

I believe in not giving up, because, in most situations, there is always something more that can be done to reduce the depth of suffering.

12

FIBROMYALGIA *BECOMES* REAL

According to legend, somewhere within the vast, creepy old cemetery that sprawls across several acres of downtown Key West, Florida, is a tombstone that reads: "I told you I was sick."

That wry posthumous sentiment is certain to resonate with the victims of fibromyalgia. For although "fibro" is not considered a fatal disease, it has forced its sufferers to justify their symptoms for hundreds of years.

A pleasant young woman whose dream was to foster children came to see me more than ten years back with complaints of chronic widespread pain. This was associated with sleep disturbances, joint stiffness, fatigue, decreased energy, and difficulty performing simple tasks. She reported worsening of pain while showering and sitting under a fan. She also reported chronic headaches. She was unable to pursue her dream because of chronic and constant pain and inability to function.

After a thorough evaluation, I diagnosed her with fibromyalgia and we discussed options for management. I told her she should mainly focus on aerobic exercise programs and change her opioid medication to duloxetine, a drug specifically approved for fibromyalgia. She was very receptive to the idea, as her life had been almost devastated by her condition and nothing seemed to work. However, there was a hitch. Her insurance company did not approve the medication. I appealed and appealed and appealed. They suggested the same medications that she had tried multiple times. After much arguing back and forth, the drug was finally approved.

The patient started noticing relief in the first two to four weeks and had significant improvement in four to six weeks, which is still continuing. She has not needed any opioid or other medications. This improvement in symptoms has allowed her to stay functional and pursue her passion of fostering children in her home. In the last ten years, she has fostered more than a dozen children who went on to finish college and start their own lives.

In her book, *The Pain Chronicles*, Melanie Thernstrom noted:

> Of the dozens of women I saw in pain clinics during my research who were suffering from fibromyalgia, every one had the experience of being disbelieved and being asked questions such as "Are you having marital problems?" in an insinuating tone, as if that was the cause of the pain. (And many were: chronic disease usually causes marital problems.)[1]

It's true that the majority, up to 75 percent, of those diagnosed with fibromyalgia are women, but it's unclear whether this is a matter of gender-based physiology or cultural conditioning. Since the symptoms are often so diffuse, some men might not feel comfortable reporting them to a doctor.

Meanwhile, although it is safe to say that fibromyalgia has been largely accepted by the medical community as a legitimate and definable condition, Dr. Daniel Clauw of the University of Michigan, heralded as an expert on the field, points out that "in many cases, people will see an average of six to eight physicians before they are ultimately diagnosed with fibromyalgia."[2]

Most of us have experienced some of the symptoms of fibromyalgia under specific circumstances. Think of how you might feel the day after an exhausting few hours spent exercising muscles you don't normally use. That overall soreness and fatigue is what fibromyalgia patients experience on a regular basis, only much worse.

On her blog, *Cassie's Site*, Cassie Osborne writes of her experience with the disease:

> On a bad day, I wake up and hurt all over. My head might hurt, it might not. My thoughts are a jumble, and I can't remember what I went into a particular room for. My hands and arms will hurt, as well as my back. The bottoms of my feet will feel like pin cushions when I

walk. My wrists will feel like I have a tight rope around them, and it seems my fingers hurt at every joint. If I'm lucky, my stomach will not hurt, but 90 percent of the time I am doubled over from the pain.[3]

No wonder many doctors feel somewhat overwhelmed when a new patient reports this onrush of seemingly unrelated symptoms. Why would a person's stomach and finger joints hurt at the same time? What would cause simultaneous headache and fatigue? Given the pressure placed on overworked general practitioners to solve problems and move on, the temptation might be to gather all of these complaints into one basket and call them "stress related." Or, perhaps, the result of a particularly virulent virus.

Eventually, many of these patients wind up coming to a pain doctor like me. What I've learned over the years is that if the tests for more easily definable ailments all come up negative, fibromyalgia must be seriously considered as the culprit. The experience of Julie Wendell is typical. As she wrote on the website ADiseaseADay.com:

> One afternoon in April 2008, after I got off work and picked up my kids, I couldn't get home fast enough. My body was overwhelmed with pain like I'd never felt before. As soon as we walked through the door, I immediately headed for the couch, where I spent the next four days.[4]

Among other things, Wendell was beset by "oppressive chest pain, muscles and joints that felt bruised, extreme coldness in my arms and face and TMJ-like jaw pain. I also had the sensation that my aching spine and pelvis were going to slide out of my body. I tried heating pads, ice packs, Tylenol and Advil, but nothing remotely helped me."[5]

Her mother, a registered nurse, first came to the conclusion that Wendell was being attacked by a flu-like virus. But her temperature was normal. Her regular physician tested her for rheumatoid arthritis, lupus, mononucleosis, and multiple sclerosis, but all those tests came back negative. Fibromyalgia was the only thing left.

But why? Why was this previously healthy individual suddenly assailed by these myriad symptoms? What causes fibromyalgia?

No one really knows, although theories abound. One is that fibromyalgia sufferers have a shortage of the natural pain reliever serotonin, which makes them more sensitive to any kind of painful stimulus. This, in turn, could be triggered by a lack of deep, healthy sleep.

Still, while that might explain how someone like Cassie Osborne or Julie Wendell might feel heightened discomfort in one part of their body, why would they suddenly experience multiple painful assaults at once?

This leads to another theory, which is that fibro, like RSD and other chronic pain afflictions, has to do with misdirected or "stuck" signals from the brain. It is as if that critical operations center were to suddenly become a paranoid schizophrenic and sense dangerous pain signals everywhere, even where none existed.

In some cases, fibromyalgia seems to "piggyback" on other diseases such as lupus and rheumatoid arthritis, to the point where it becomes almost impossible to tell where one stops and the other begins. The connection with lupus has sent some researchers off in the direction of possible autoimmune deficiency.

As reported by a popular fibromyalgia website:

> Factors perceived to worsen these symptoms included emotional distress (83% frequency), weather changes (80%), sleeping problems (79%), strenuous activity (70%), mental stress (68%), worrying (60%), car travel (57%), family conflicts (52%), and physical injuries and physical inactivity (both at 50%), among others. The trigger most frequently cited as leading to the onset of fibromyalgia was chronic stress (41.9%), followed by emotional trauma (31.3%), acute illness (26.7%), physical injury (non-motor vehicle related; 17.1%), and surgery and motor vehicle accident (both at 16.1%). Just over 20% of respondents stated that they could not identify any particular triggering event for the onset of their fibromyalgia.[6]

The most elusive quarry for an ever-increasing group of researchers is a "silver bullet" symptom that would be common to everyone with fibromyalgia. So far, the closest anyone has come is identifying a collection of "trigger points" that seem to be hypersensitive.

Dr. Muhammad Yunus of the Illinois College of Medicine has researched fibromyalgia extensively and has made some preliminary links to the human leukocyte antigen gene.[7] Daniel Clauw also believes that at least some aspects of fibromyalgia might be hereditary.

Furthermore, Dr. Yunus wants to remove the condition as a stand-alone disease and group it with other neurological conditions, such as chronic fatigue syndrome and myofascial pain syndrome. These overlap with fibro to the point where many consider them the same disease. He would call the new classification *central sensitivity syndromes.* [8]

Of central sensitivity syndrome, or CSS, it is said:

> CSS is not the cause of fibromyalgia, it is a decided factor in the persistent pain. CS is believed to start when persistent pain signaling (nerves telling body it hurts) causes cells in the spinal cord to become over-activated. The pain-transmitting cells become more sensitive as a result which causes stimuli that would normally be perceived as mildly painful to be perceived instead as extremely painful. Even a light touch can be perceived as very painful—an effect called allodynia. [9]

But despite all the research that is being done on fibromyalgia, there are still going to be people who are skeptical of the condition.

This raises the question: What would be the advantage for someone faking fibromyalgia? Disability pay is almost always less than regular pay, and most chronic ailments would far outlast that regular check. The drugs generally used to combat fibromyalgia rarely include any of the opioid family (the drugs most likely to be abused for pleasure). The drugs most likely to be prescribed are basic analgesics, sedatives for sleep, and antidepressants such as Prozac and Paxil (and, most recently, Lyrica and Cymbalta).

If someone wanted to obtain any of the latter drugs by deception, it would be much easier to feign depression, not fibromyalgia. And finally, most pain doctors require strict medication accountability from their patients—no fun likely there.

Dr. John Kissel of the Ohio State University Medical Center said in an article published by the American Academy of Neurology that he was originally a fibromyalgia doubter.

> Then he saw patients that began to change his mind. He still remembers one woman in her 40s, a professional trial attorney from Columbus, OH. She had developed debilitating fatigue and horrible muscle pain and tenderness about a month after getting over a mild case of the flu.

"After performing a number of tests," Kissell said, "I went in to speak with her and mentioned fibromyalgia. She asked, 'What's that?' I said, 'You haven't heard of fibromyalgia? People are talking about it all over the place.' She said to me, 'I work 14 hours a day as a trial attorney—I don't do outside reading.' She wasn't depressed. She was still working. But she had all the typical symptoms of fibromyalgia. That was a formative experience in my thinking about the condition."[10]

In the past, Kissel said, there had been legitimate reasons for skepticism about fibromyalgia:

> The majority of research in fibromyalgia was not adequate. Studies would pick some parameter and look at it only in patients with fibromyalgia and sometimes in normal controls, without comparing them to people with other chronic pain conditions, patients with depression, or to patients with other muscle diseases.
>
> What's more, some physicians tended to view it as a grab-bag condition, diagnosed only when the doctor couldn't find anything else. Patients would come in and say, "I have muscle pain." The doctor would do all kinds of tests—electromyography (a test for abnormal electrical activity in the muscles), blood work, muscle biopsies, and imaging, and if all that was negative, then voilà, it was fibromyalgia.[11]

Indeed, the relationship between conventional medicine and fibromyalgia has followed something of a bell curve path. First, it was discounted. Then, it was embraced. Now, as more and more fibromyalgia sufferers take their misery to us, hoping to be healed, we are learning that the more we uncover about their condition, the more perplexing it becomes.

We now acknowledge that fibromyalgia is not simply a phantom ailment restricted to hypochondriacs, a "somatic" will of the wisp conjured up by emotional turmoil. These patients hurt, and we can tell that they hurt. We know that you can't catch fibromyalgia, although you may inherit it. We don't understand the variances in symptoms from one individual to another, nor its relationship with similar conditions such as lupus and rheumatoid arthritis.

There are, however, those trigger points.

About the size of a penny, trigger points are sensitive areas just below the skin, generally located around the joints. They often *seem* to be inflamed, and yet closer examination usually shows no inflammation. Eighteen of these points have been identified, occurring in the same general areas with every individual. Trigger points are tested by gentle probing with an instrument known as a dosimeter and often compared to nontender points to make sure the painful reaction is not just limited to those areas.[12]

Might these be tiny keys to unlocking the mystery of fibromyalgia, or are they as irrelevant as the spots on the skin of someone with measles? We don't know yet.

In the end, until more research gives us a clear diagnostic test or some other reliable means of arriving at fibromyalgia as the cause of a patient's pain, we will have to deal with that pain on a surface level, confronting whatever symptoms present themselves and setting aside the mystery until later. In other words, we are learning to match the treatment to the individual, wherever the pain comes from.

At the same time, we're also beginning to include physical therapy and counseling and even some alternative healing modalities in an effort to treat the whole person. For it is the whole person that conditions like fibromyalgia attack—and we want that person back.

13

OTHER PAIN CONDITIONS

WORST PAIN CULPRITS

A complete list of the illnesses, injuries, and brain-body malfunctions that have been known to cause chronic pain would overflow this chapter and hopelessly confuse the reader.

Some are familiar to many: osteoarthritis, lupus, Lyme disease, multiple sclerosis, spinal injuries, and migraine headaches, to name a few.

Many of the conditions that cause chronic pain can fit in two broad categories: those that cause nociceptive pain and those resulting in neuropathic pain. Many more have a mix of these features.

The nociceptive pain occurs when the receptors in the body detect potentially noxious or harmful stimuli. In contrast, neuropathic pain results from involvement of peripheral or central nervous tissue. The two pain types are felt differently. The nociceptive pain is usually the sharp, throbbing pain that we feel when we accidently cut our finger with a blade. In contrast, neuropathic pain is described as the burning or shooting pain that a patient with neuropathy from diabetes may complain about. In spite of extensive research, the exact mechanism of neuropathic pain is still not very clear. And when something is not very clear, there are theories.

An article in *European Neuropsychopharmacology* suggests that "several maladaptive mechanisms underlying these symptoms have been elucidated in recent years: peripheral sensitization of nociception, abnormal excitability of afferent neurons, central sensitization comprising pronociceptive facilitation, disinhibition of nociception and central reorganization processes, and sympathetically maintained pain."[1]

Neuropathic pain is a predominant feature of multiple conditions that afflict the human body. The classic examples are postherpetic neuralgia (PHN), reflex sympathetic dystrophy (RSD)/complex regional pain syndrome (CRPS), diabetes, migraines, and postamputation phantom limb pain.

Reflex Sympathetic Dystrophy/Complex Regional Pain Syndrome

A twenty-one-year-old man who worked as a landscaper had an accident in which he injured his right foot and ankle. He had broken bones and underwent surgery to fix these. The surgery went well, but the pain did not improve. In the coming weeks and months, the pain went from bad to worse, to the extent that he had to stop working altogether. He was on multiple medications, including heavy opioids, when I first saw him. A detailed history, a thorough evaluation, and further testing revealed CRPS. I offered and discussed a multipronged approach, including aggressive physical therapy and a trial of lumbar sympathetic blocks. The patient was initially hesitant, but when the pain became unbearable, he agreed to the plan. I performed a series of blocks, and he noticed relief starting with the first block. By the end of the series, his pain had improved considerably, he noticed warming of his leg and foot and the ability to bear weight and function to an almost normal level. This happened two years back, and the patient has not needed to consult us for further management since.

This is an illustration of a very positive result from an early diagnosis and management. Most patients are not that lucky and suffer with excruciating pain for years.

CRPS, as illustrated above, and postherpetic neuralgia (PHN) are two of the worst offenders on the "chronic pain causing" list. As a pain doctor, I can vouch for the evil reputations of both.

First, RSD/CRPS and PHN are often excruciatingly painful. PHN, while not life threatening in the usual sense, has driven patients to suicide because they couldn't imagine sharing their lives any longer with pain of that intensity. RSD combines pain with muscle and tissue damage that can be irreversible and can result in complete loss of function of the limb.

From a doctor's perspective, these are also two of the most difficult conditions to isolate and treat. This is especially true with RSD/CRPS.

Like phantom limb syndrome, where an amputee still feels pain or some other sensation where the amputated limb used to be, RSD/CRPS might be described as the inappropriate aftermath to an injury of a nerve or soft tissue. This reaction can be far out of proportion to the seriousness of the wound and often continues long after the initial trauma seems to be healed.

> RSD most commonly occurs in the four extremities but some people have it in other areas such as eyes, ears, back, face, etc. What does it feel like? Well, if you had it in your hand, imagine your hand was doused in gasoline, lit on fire, and then kept that way 24 hours a day, 7 days a week, and you knew it was never going to be put out. Now imagine it both hands, arms, legs, feet, eyes, ears; well, you get the picture. I sometimes sit there and am amazed that no one else can see the flames shooting off of my body.
>
> The second component to CRPS is what is called Allodynia. Allodynia is an extreme sensitivity to touch, sound, and/or vibration. Imagine that same hand now has the skin all burned off and is completely raw. Next, rub some salt on top of it and then rub some sandpaper on top of that! THAT is allodynia! Picture getting pretty vivid? Now, because of the allodynia, any normal touch will cause pain; your clothing, the gentle touch of a loved one, a sheet, rain, shower, razor, hairbrush, shoe, someone brushing by you in a crowded hallway, etc. In addition, sounds, especially loud or deep sounds and vibrations, will also cause pain; a school bell, thunder, loud music, crowds, singing, yelling, sirens, traffic, kids screaming, loud wind, even the sound in a typical movie theatre. This is what allodynia is all about. Imagine going through your daily life where everything that you touch, or that touches you, where most every noise around you from a passing car or plane to children playing, causes you pain, this, in addition to the enormous pain you are already experiencing from the CRPS itself.[2]

RSD/CRPS can also produce inflammation, increased sweating, skin rashes, low-grade fever, sores, insomnia and memory loss.[3]

As you can see, because of the various symptoms, RSD/CRPS can be very difficult to diagnose. To borrow from the old parable, doctors can become like blind men and the patient is the elephant. Depending on the emphasis, this condition can resemble fibromyalgia, PHN, carpal tunnel syndrome, Lyme disease, or any of a dozen other ailments.

A few windows into RSD/CRPS have been recently opened for physicians, however. Unlike some other mysterious and invisible nerve conditions that cause chronic pain, RSD often makes its presence obvious—not just to scans and X-rays but to the naked eye. The skin can turn various colors (blue, black, red) and become shiny. The affected area can become cold to the touch. Tissues can swell. Bones can be compromised to the point where they become osteoporotic and deformed.

If nothing else, this can be advantageous to a patient who is planning to petition for disability or is asking for compensation for a previous injury. According to the RSD Foundation,

> Many patients who develop RSD/CRPS as the result of an injury do so within the context of legal liability. Some patients can be expected to defend their rights in courts of law. It is not uncommon for the defendant to accuse the patient of faking their condition, especially if there are no objective findings of RSD/CRPS documented on the medical record.
>
> Therefore, the attending physician must assess more than just subjective complaints (medical history). The physician must aggressively seek and document [more obvious symptoms]. For example, about 80 percent of RSD/CRPS cases have differences in temperature in opposite sides that may be colder or warmer. These temperature changes may be associated with changes in skin color. Furthermore, the temperature differences are not just static. The skin temperature can undergo dynamic changes in a relatively short period of time (within minutes).[4]

Thus, the most effective aid in proving the existence of RSD/CRPS may be one of the oldest in the doctor's tool bag—the humble thermometer.

Yet how to proceed once a diagnosis is made is another challenge altogether. RSD can dispatch discomfort to odd parts of the body, often considerably removed from the original injury. It can destroy bone, freeze a shoulder, lock a hand into a fist. It can spread from an arm to the face and vice versa.

The RSD Foundation's *Reflex Sympathetic Dystrophy Clinical Practice Guidelines* provides this explanation:

> For reasons we do not understand, in individuals who go on to develop RSD/CRPS, the central nervous system appears to assume an abnormal function. Theoretically, this sympathetic activity at the site of injury could cause an inflammatory response, causing the blood vessels to spasm, leading to more swelling and pain. The events could lead to more pain, triggering another response, establishing a vicious cycle of pain.[5]

No one wants to have the phrase "for reasons we do not understand" attached to a description of their condition. But while RSD is said to occur in from 5 to 7 percent of all traumatic injuries, especially fractures, it has been largely marginalized by the medical profession.

Whenever we call something a *complex*, it usually means that we don't get it. Is RSD/CRPS a self-contained disease or condition with diverse symptoms, or is it a vague collection of unrelated symptoms that we group together only for the sake of medical convenience?

Hawaii resident Tina Mohr offered another possible meaning for the letters "RSD": really scary disease.

Mohr's RSD experience began with a bad fall—a slip on some soapy water on a sidewalk. She tore a ligament in her left knee and received an ugly abrasion on her left elbow. A few weeks after the incident, following knee surgery, things began to get strange.

"I was at a restaurant with my family," Mohr recalled.

> I picked up a glass of ice water with my left hand. A stinging cold pain made me put down the glass immediately. . . . I picked up the glass with my right hand but it felt a "normal" cold. I touched the glass again with my left hand, "Wow!" I said again! The glass felt so much colder to my left hand than my right. It actually hurt to hold the glass in my left hand.
>
> A couple of days later, I was in the shower. I leaned to my right. "Whoa!" The water got burning hot. "Who flushed a toilet in the other bathroom?" I thought. . . . Soon I leaned back into the water and it felt "normal" hot again. After leaning to the left and to the right a few times in succession, I realized that the left side of my body perceived the water to be much hotter than the right side.[6]

At first, Mohr just regarded these incidents as quirky. But then . . .

> One night near the end of that week at 3 am, I awoke with a star-
> tle. . . . . It felt as though something on my left arm was crawling and
> burning. There was a deep, almost throbbing and fiery ache in my
> arm. It was very painful. Then a breeze crept in through the window
> by my bed and immediately accentuated the pain. In a drowsy daze,
> I thought, "Boy, this is just like RSD."[7]

Mohr had studied RSD in massage school. Later, in her massage practice, she had worked on a woman who suffered from the condition and
needed a morphine pump.

"Then, I couldn't even fathom her pain," Mohr wrote.

Indeed, every RSD case is different. Mohr not only watched in hor-
ror as her left forearm shrunk noticeably, but she experienced a series
of small seizures. Meanwhile, the sensitivity to temperature in the affected area only grew more pronounced.

"By the winter of 2000," she said,

> I learned I slept best with my left arm in my down jacket and my left
> hand protected by a winter glove. Hawaii winters are relatively
> warm, but my left arm and hand found even the slightest rumination
> of a whisper-cool breeze to be unbearable and my arm and hand
> begged to be well protected. The intrinsic muscles in my left arm
> atrophied and my hand felt clumsy.
>
> Initially, I was sent to an arm specialist who X-rayed my elbow.
> He advised SSEP nerve conduction testing and a cervical MRI. The
> nerve conduction testing of both left extremities (arm and leg) came
> out normal. My cervical MRI showed problems, but they did not
> exactly correlate to the subtle atrophic changes in my left hand.[8]

Derrick Phillips, founder of the RSD alert site, also tracks his problems back to a fall. It happened while he was hiking the mountains of
his native Britain and broke his left arm, which ultimately led to paralysis in his left hand.

"Paralysis is ignored in the new medical name for the condition
(Chronic Regional Pain Syndrome)," he wrote, "but in my case, it is a
key factor. Over the years, I found that if I stopped exercising my hand,
it would start to stiffen up and I would get twinges that weren't quite
pain."[9]

At one point, Phillips related, he was unable to move his left index finger.

Most physicians agree that it is important to make a diagnosis of RSD/CRPS in its early incarnation. The Cleveland Clinic has gathered a synopsis of symptoms in three semidefinable stages, and stage three in this version is grim indeed.

1. Severe bone, muscle and skin damage: the changes in affected bone, muscles and skin become irreversible. The skin becomes tight and muscle and other tissue becomes weak and constricted.
2. Constant pain: The pain becomes unyielding (although for some, the pain decreases in stage three).
3. Severe mobility limitations: There is a muscle atrophy and severely limited mobility of the affected area. Joint movement is greatly impaired and occasionally the limb will be displaced from its normal position. [10]

As mentioned earlier, however, early diagnosis can only be achieved after ruling out the myriad other conditions, aspects of which RSD/CRPS might mimic. By the time a patient has been through a series of general practitioners and down a number of diagnostic dead ends, the clock has already been ticking.

Diagnosis is not a problem for postherpetic neuralgia, however. Unlike RSD/CRPS, which often seems to choose its victims at random, PHN is directly tied to another disease, chicken pox.

In fact, the two share the same varicella zoster virus. In some cases, instead of fading away after causing chicken pox, this virus will take refuge in nerve tissue and lurk there for years. If it reappears, it's often with a vengeance.

The more fortunate victims of this second stage of the virus develop shingles, which is bad enough. It generally arrives with the flu-like symptoms of headache, fever, and upper respiratory distress. It then lays down a rash—often on the chest but also on the back and face. It then commonly mutates into water-filled blisters that can leave their owner feeling like the Elephant Man. If it gets into the eyes, it can cause blindness. The only good thing about shingles is that it, like chicken pox, generally goes away. Unless the patient is elderly or has a weakened immune system from conditions like cancer or is simply unlucky. That's when PHN sets in, a malevolent echo of shingles damage to nerve endings. As with other chronic pain afflictions, the body doesn't seem to realize that the varicella zoster infection is gone.

Roughly one in five people with shingles later contracts PHN, mostly those over fifty (a more than 50 percent chance). If you manage to reach the age of eighty, avoid chicken pox and shingles at all costs. In the eighty-and-older age group, PHN follows shingles in 80 percent of the cases.

In terms of symptoms, PHN is often described by those it torments as "the chicken pox from hell." It burns, it aches, and it itches. The viral assault often leaves the skin highly sensitive to touch or pressure—even a breeze.

Drugs generally prescribed for PHN include tricyclic antidepressants, steroids, anticonvulsants, and in cases of extreme pain, opioids. There is, I should add, considerable disagreement among pain specialists as to whether the latter class of drugs works on neuropathic pain.

A Florida-based pain specialist named Andrea Trescot has made a crusade of educating family physicians about the need to intervene with shingles patients—especially the elderly—before PHN gains a foothold. She writes:

> As the US population ages, the incidence of shingles (and therefore post herpetic neuralgia) would be expected to increase. However, the expected increased utilization of medical resources can be significant, both initially and long term. Early interventional treatment is effective and provides rapid and often complete relief.
>
> Because of the time issues, it is critical that patients and physicians be educated in the importance of rapid and aggressive treatment. Too often, patients are told that "nothing can be done" and that "the rash will go away on its own." Unfortunately, pain physicians are usually used to seeing chronic pain patients, where onset of treatment is not an issue. It is not uncommon for many pain practices to have 4 to 6 week waiting times for an appointment, clearly too long to wait with this condition.
>
> Community doctors have to be educated by the pain practitioners themselves regarding the acute interventional treatment of shingles. In our practice, we lecture frequently to the family doctors in my area, explaining to them the "code word"—"active shingles"—which will get their patient in my office that day or the next morning. [11]

The pattern that repeatedly emerges in this chapter is that early detection and aggressive management is the key. The excruciating pain and suffering that accompanies these conditions can wither even the bravest.

Cesare Pavese, an Italian poet and author, may not have been thinking of RSD/CRPS or PHN, but his description illustrates these conditions well:

> Suffering is by no means a privilege, a sign of nobility, a reminder of God. Suffering is a fierce, bestial thing, commonplace, uncalled for, natural as air. It is intangible; no one can grasp it or fight against it; it dwells in time—is the same thing as time; if it comes in fits and starts, that is only so as to leave the sufferer more defenseless during the moments that follow, those long moments when one relives the last bout of torture and waits for the next. [12]

OTHER CONDITIONS

In the previous section, we discussed conditions that often lead to agonizing pain. There are other varied conditions that also result in chronic pain. Considerable research has been done toward understanding of many of them, but some are still a mystery.

Multiple Sclerosis

It is a potentially disabling disease of the brain and spinal cord (central nervous system).

In MS, the immune system attacks the protective sheath (myelin) that covers nerve fibers and causes communication problems between your brain and the rest of your body. Eventually, the disease can cause the nerves themselves to deteriorate or become permanently damaged.

Signs and symptoms of MS vary widely and depend on the amount of nerve damage and which nerves are affected. Some people with severe MS may lose the ability to walk independently or at all, while others may experience long periods of remission without any new symptoms.

There's no cure for multiple sclerosis. However, treatments can help speed recovery from attacks, modify the course of the disease and manage symptoms.[13]

In a study titled "Chronic Pain in Multiple Sclerosis: Is There Also Fibromyalgia?"[14] the authors report:

Pain is a common and disabling symptom in persons with multiple sclerosis (MS), with a prevalence ranging widely between 29% and 86%. Several different pain conditions are associated with MS and may be defined by location, by presumed mechanism, and by duration, ranging from paroxysmal to chronic. Restricting our focus to chronic pain, approximately 75% of MS patients report having had pain within 1 month prior to assessment. One broad category of MS-related pain is central neuropathic pain, which includes dysesthetic extremity pain, a chronic form of pain described as the most common. Other chronic pain conditions are musculoskeletal pain (e.g., back pain), painful tonic spasms, and headache.[15]

Phantom Limb Pain Syndrome

Phantom limb pain syndrome is a condition where patients feel that the amputated limb, or other organ, is still attached. This is fairly common. However, a small proportion feel persistent pain in the amputated limb. This is a classic example of neuropathic pain and one that can be very hard to manage.

Multiple factors including site of amputation or presence of preamputation pain have been found to have a positive correlation with the development of phantom limb pain. The paradigms of proposed mechanisms have shifted over the past years from the psychogenic theory to peripheral and central neural changes involving cortical reorganization. More recently, the role of mirror neurons in the brain has been proposed in the generation of phantom pain.[16]

Treatment options for phantom limb pain include nerve pain medications like gabapentin and antidepressants, interventional procedures like epidural injections, physical and psychotherapy, psychobehavioral techniques like a mirror box, and pain modulation through implanted stimulators.

Even with such options, the cure is usually elusive.

Migraines

Migraines are headaches, usually familial, many times one sided and sometimes associated with other symptoms, that affect a considerable portion of our society. They result in significant loss of functional hours. Attacks may be followed by a postdromal period when patients may be dizzy, drowsy, or confused. Attacks may be associated with aura. These are sensations that patients may see, smell, feel, or experience, usually before an attack.

A paper in *Therapeutic Advances of Chronic Disease* describes that there are three broad approaches to treating chronic migraines: lifestyle and trigger management, acute treatments (i.e., those taken during attacks or exacerbations of chronic pain), and preventive treatments (medication or other interventions designed to reduce the tendency to have attacks). While many patients find that lifestyle adjustments such as regularizing meals and sleep can reduce the frequency of their attacks, some form of medication or other treatment is almost invariably necessary in patients with chronic migraine.[17]

As a young man, one of my favorite quotes was from Aristotle, "The more you know, the more you know you don't know."

That is as much true for anything else as it is for chronic pain.

14

GETTING MOVING—EXERCISE AND PHYSICAL THERAPY

EXERCISE: THE MIRACLE CURE

Two years back, the Academy of Medical Royal Colleges (AOMRC) came out with an extensive report[1] on the beneficial effects of exercise deduced on the basis of the most recent scientific information. The report also laid out guidelines on how physicians, and other providers, can implement these findings to help change the lives of their patients. They called it "the Miracle Cure."

We in the scientific community have long known that exercise and regular physical activity have positive effects on such varied conditions as obesity, diabetes, heart disease, and high cholesterol. In fact, we have promoted this avenue with other modalities like medications for decades.

What is new is the sheer amount of evidence-based literature that has been released recently showing that these effects are much more pronounced and have an effect on many more areas, and the recommendation is that exercise be incorporated in most management plans.

The AOMRC report, in this review of the latest evidence, says that the four most proximate causes of illness include smoking, poor nutrition, lack of physical activity, and alcohol excess. Of these, the importance of regular exercise is the least well known. The recommendation is for at least five days of thirty minutes of moderate exercise. It has to

be at least moderate—enough to get a person slightly out of breath and/
or sweaty and to increase the heart rate.

We now know that moderate exercise provides up to 30 percent
improvement in the conditions described above, as well as in depression, dementia, and some cancers. It also can reduce the chances of
premature death and long-term diseases.

The health improvements with regular physical activity are often
greater than many drugs.[2]

The AOMRC reports mounting evidence that physical inactivity is a
major causative physical link between social inequality and poor health.
There is economic evidence for focusing on increasing physical activity
as a means of improving health and reducing inequalities in health care.

The academy advises doctors that they may need to reassure people
that the risks of exercise are very low. For example, the risks of sudden
death or severe cardiac events during exercise are extremely rare. Many
activities can be promoted: brisk walking, cycling, climbing stairs, dog
walking, using outdoor gyms, and dancing—even sexual activity can
bring some benefits. Basing activities in communities leads to sustained
acceptance.

Another paper looked at exercise in the treatment of pain. It concludes that "exercise is effective for the management of chronic low
back pain for up to 1 year after treatment and for fibromyalgia syndrome for up to 6 months (level 2). There is conflicting evidence (level
4b) about which exercise program is effective for chronic low back pain.
For chronic neck pain and for chronic soft tissue shoulder disorders and
chronic lateral epicondylitis, evidence of effectiveness of exercise is
limited (level 3)."[3]

In November 2016, the American Cancer Society reported that
more than four in ten cancers and cancer deaths are linked to modifiable risk factors. Two of the important factors are obesity and physical
inactivity. Other significant factors include smoking, drinking, eating
red or processed meats, ultraviolet radiation, and cancer-associated in-
fections.

Further, the report estimates that physical inactivity contributed to
26.7 percent of uterine cancers, 16.3 percent of colorectal cancers, and
3.9 percent of female breast cancers.[4]

[A] study investigated associations between frequency, duration, and intensity of recreational exercise and chronic pain in a cross-sectional survey of the adult population of a Norwegian county (the Nord-Trøndelag Health Study; HUNT 3). Of the 94,194 invited to participate, complete data were obtained from 46,533 participants. Separate analyses were performed for the working-age population (20–64 years) and the older population (65 years or more). When defined as pain lasting longer than 6 months, and of at least moderate intensity during the past month, the overall prevalence of chronic pain was 29%. We found that increased frequency, duration, and intensity of exercise were associated with less chronic pain in analyses adjusted for age, education, and smoking. For those aged 20–64 years, the prevalence of chronic pain was 10–12% lower for those exercising 1–3 times a week for at least 30 minutes duration or of moderate intensity, relative to those not exercising. Dependent on the load of exercise, the prevalence of chronic pain was 21–38% lower among older women who exercised, relative to those not exercising. Similar, but somewhat weaker, associations were seen for older men. This study shows consistent and linear associations between frequency, duration, and intensity of recreational exercise and chronic pain for the older population, and associations without apparent linear shape for the working-age population.[5]

My favorite pastime is running. I try to get in fifteen to twenty miles a week, and I have run most of the ten-mile races in our town. Every year, my main goal is to beat my previous year's record by at least one minute. And many years I have accomplished this goal. I keep my medals in my office in clear view of my patients so that they will notice and, hopefully, start a discussion. This is a cue for me to seize the occasion and guide them toward a plan of action of their own.

The role of exercise and activity on physical well-being, and obesity in general and chronic pain in particular, is significant.

My patients offer me an opportunity to share their health concerns, and I take every such opportunity to guide them toward a more active and healthy lifestyle.

Sometimes it is harder for healthy people to consider increasing their physical activity and indulge in a regular exercise program because they think that they do not need it. Once affected by a musculoskeletal condition that affects their quality of life, they may be more prone to accept physical therapy as a significant part of their management plan.

This brings us to the next section of this chapter.

FIGHTING BACK WITH PHYSICAL THERAPY

Wildlife experts tell us that the best course of action when attacked by a grizzly bear is to fall down, curl into a fetal position, and play dead.

As tempting as it might seem, however, this is not the way to deal with an attack of chronic pain.

Especially as we get older, our muscles react badly to periods of inaction. In the world of chronic pain, a prime example of this is reflex sympathetic dystrophy/complex regional pain syndrome (RSD/CRPS), where an inability to use the limb results in a vicious circle of loss of limb function from severe muscle atrophy and osteoporosis.

Fortunately, most chronic pain afflictions are not that ferocious. Still, medical science has been moving steadily away from the old advice "better stay off that until it heals."

It is, of course, important to draw a distinction here between acute and chronic pain. Naturally, a serious wound or fracture or major surgery requires a period of convalescence. However, even in many of those cases, hospital patients are surprised when they are rousted out of bed and told to walk the halls within days of their trauma.

Therefore, meet the new, old mantra: Use it or lose it.

As with all medical trends, this one has been approaching for a while. Back in November 1998, the journal of the International Association for the Study of Pain reported:

> Health care has changed in recent decades. Early activity for recovery of function is now encouraged, and the impairment model has broadened to include psychosocial components. A multidisciplinary team approach now includes the person as an educated and active participant, and physical therapy treatments emphasize activity. The therapist's role has changed from healer to helper. Therapists help patients address and overcome physical and psychological obstacles, return to activities, and achieve personal goals.[6]

I would much rather write a prescription for physical therapy than medication, although I certainly understand the importance of the latter in some situations. Chronic pain can be soul and mind crushing, and even the most stoic of patients can be beaten down over time. With no apparent end in sight, they begin to slide slowly into the toxic attitude of "Why me? What did I do to deserve this?"

Without question, many of these people have every reason to feel sorry for themselves. Unfortunately, that's counterproductive.

Right after I finished my fellowship training at the University of Virginia and started practicing pain medicine, I noticed severe pain in my right shoulder. I did not have any obvious injury, but the pain was excruciating. My range of motion had greatly diminished. I couldn't move my arm away from my body or lift it up in front of me. In the office, my seasoned nurse recommended physical therapy. Back at the university, my other fellows and I had discussed physical therapy and whether or not it was more of a placebo effect than an actual management option. Accordingly, I hesitated. When the pain started getting worse in the next week, I went to see my neighborhood physical therapist. I still wasn't convinced that this would do any good, but I wanted to give it a try. She examined me, printed a schedule of exercise programs, and gave me a pink and a blue rubber band to work with. This made me even more reluctant to start the program. I went home and decided to go ahead with the exercises anyway. I felt soreness and pressure while doing the exercises, and the pain started to disappear over the course of the next few days. By the end of the week, I had no pain and had completely restored my shoulder's range of motion and strength back to normal without a single pill. Suddenly, I was a believer in physical therapy. Since then, this option has been a predominant and reliable approach for many of my pain patients. Most of the musculoskeletal disorders benefit from an aggressive course of physical therapy and a continued home exercise plan.

Some months back, a patient was referred to me for chronic low back pain. This was a seventy-year-old female with lumbar degenerative disc disease. When I first saw her in my office, I noticed that she was holding her left arm very close to her body and was unable to move it. When I asked her about it, she said that she is not worried about it because it had been like this for many years and she does not use her left arm for anything. She had pain in the left shoulder and arm and felt that it was there to stay. I discussed this issue with her and suggested that we work on this first, even when she had presented to us with back issues. She agreed to a treatment plan that consisted of anti-inflammatory medications and a series of shoulder nerve blocks, each followed immediately by an aggressive physical therapy program. Within three weeks, her range of motion in her left arm was restored to near normal and her pain had considerably improved. To this day, she continues with a home exercise plan.

Physical therapy has obvious benefits in terms of loosening, strengthening, and even reprogramming balky muscles and joints. But there are other plusses as well:

1. Exercise often makes us feel good because it releases natural endorphins.
2. If the physical therapy is out of the home, it helps the patient avoid isolation and interact with others.
3. It gives chronic pain patients a sense of fighting back—a more proactive role in managing their health.
4. Although we all think we know our bodies intimately, we aren't always tuned in to how much stress to put on them at certain times. Left to their own instincts, some chronic pain sufferers would overdo their exercise routines in their impatience to feel better. Others might be too timid to work through the pain in a positive way. The physical therapist is trained to steer his or her clients down a middle road.

For physical therapists, chronic pain patients present special challenges. When dealing with this condition, the impairment tests that physical therapists rely on can sometimes correlate poorly with a patient's dysfunction. For example, a physical therapist may test for muscle strength, range of motion, or velocity of motion to give the therapist a grasp on how to treat the patient. However, chronic pain patients may have erratic results. This is due to a couple of factors. One, the patient might be afraid of exacerbating his or her pain by straining too much and therefore may not work as hard. Two, the patient may have psychological factors that are affecting his or her assessment performance, such as depression and low perceived self-efficacy.

This is why the International Association for the Study of Pain advises that

measured performance tests are best when quick, simple and meaningful to both patient and practitioner. Those that use minimal (if any) special equipment, are inexpensive, and test functions of every-day life compromised by chronic pain have been adopted in clinical practice. Persons with pain tend to move more slowly than pain-free persons, generate less force during muscle testing, and may have poor endurance during exercise.[7]

For men, especially, this can be a heavy psychological burden. For someone who has been in good physical shape earlier in life, it can be humiliating to struggle through exercises they would have once performed with ease. This is true of active women, as well, but men have a greater tendency to base part of their identity on their physical vigor.

An "outside" person might not realize this or understand the extent to which a chronic pain sufferer might be limited—especially if the affliction is something that is not immediately noticeable.

A good physical therapist can gently guide patients into the realm of lowered expectations. A person with fibromyalgia or RSD/CRPS is not training for the Olympics but rather for the physical strength needed to mow the lawn or clean the house. Some patients might actually far exceed those expectations, but the last thing anyone with chronic pain needs is another reason to feel helpless and defeated.

Moreover, the therapist should always be working in conjunction with a physician. Before the patient arrives at the physical therapy center, the pain doctor has already worked up an assessment of his or her limitations, prognosis, and particular pain problems. The physician often lists the areas that the therapist needs to focus on. That way, the therapist can limit the often-painful initial period of exploration.

The current overall treatment trend could be described as "it takes a village to help a chronic pain patient." That "village" might include a pain physician, a physical therapist, a counselor or a dietician, and even a yoga or massage therapist, if that fits with the patient's wishes.

RSD/CRPS patients can benefit immensely from physical therapy. A study performed by Anne E. Daly and Andrea Biolacerkowski concluded:

> People with CRPS often develop guarding behaviors where they avoid using or touching the affected limb. This inactivity exacerbates the disease and perpetuates the pain cycle. Therefore, optimizing the multimodal treatment is paramount to allow for use of the involved body part. Physical therapy works best for most patients, especially

goal-directed therapy, where the patient begins from an initial point, regardless of how minimal, and then endeavors to increase activity each week.

Narrative synthesis of the results, based on effect size, found there was good to very good quality level II evidence that graded motor imagery is effective in reducing pain in adults with CRPS-1, irrespective of the outcome measure used. No evidence was found to support treatments frequently recommended in clinical guidelines, such as stress loading.[8]

In the case of RSD/CRPS patients, the slogan "No pain, no gain" can only be taken so far. In some cases, when movement is too painful for the patient to bear, it initially can be done under light anesthesia to avoid damage to atrophied tissue and bones.

With most chronic pain problems, however, physical therapy is a key factor in early intervention. The longer a person remains inactive waiting for a diagnosis, the more difficult it may be to redeem parts of the body that have lost their function.

It is important to remember that physical therapy also has a "passive" side that may include massage or the use of a number of different machines to stimulate muscles. A significant part of the plan includes the "homework" to be done between appointments and continued after in-office appointments end.

As public knowledge of chronic pain increases, many practitioners of yoga, tai chi, reiki (a form of relaxation therapy using heat from the hands but not actual touch), and massage have developed specific programs to address it. Many YMCAs and gyms around the country have also taken notice, offering low-impact exercise regimes.

A 2008 study found that aquatic exercise was especially beneficial in countering the effects of fibromyalgia. As reported in the *Washington Post* in 2008:

> The study from the University of Extremadura in Spain and the University of Evora, Portugal, included 33 women with fibromyalgia—17 did supervised one-hour exercise sessions in a heated pool three times a week for eight months, while the other 16 did no aquatic training.
>
> The researchers found that the long-term aquatic exercise helped reduce fibromyalgia symptoms and improved the women's health-related quality of life. In an earlier study, the same researchers found

that a short-term exercise program helped ease symptoms, but pain returned when patients completed the exercise regimen.

"The addition of an aquatic exercise program to the usual care for fibromyalgia in women is cost-effective in terms of both health care costs and societal costs," and "appropriate aquatic exercise is a good health investment," the researchers wrote.[9]

Range of motion can considerably improve in water, and the increased resistance can be used for strength training. Performing these activities in a heated pool can have the additional benefit of increasing the blood supply to the area and improving healing.

For most people, a regular schedule of aerobic exercise and a strength training routine is essential for maintaining form and function. In those with moderate chronic pain, regular walking affords major benefits. As with everything else, let your body be your guide as to how far to go.

Whether or not you choose to do physical therapy, yoga, tai chi, reiki, or massage, getting proactive about your health can help you feel empowered again.

For nothing influences our body and mind more than the thought of being in control.

15

INTERVENTIONAL PAIN MANAGEMENT

CONVENTIONAL APPROACHES

> The expectations of life depend upon diligence; the mechanic that
> would perfect his work must first sharpen his tools.
>
> —Confucius

Whether someone is a chronic pain sufferer or a physician trying to ease that pain, instant gratification can be elusive. To me, that's the most rewarding aspect of nerve blocks, ablation procedures, and peripheral nerve and spinal cord stimulation. When they work, they often work quickly.

An interventional pain physician's main armamentarium includes a wide variety of procedures in his tool box. We use these as part of a comprehensive management plan. Many times, other options are used simultaneously, including physical therapy, psychological help, and medications.

Let's return for a moment to Melanie Thernstrom's vivid metaphor of neuropathic pain as a security alarm that refuses to turn off. With a security alarm, the homeowner will find some way to disconnect the device, either temporarily or permanently. Some nerve blocks, ablation procedures, and neuromodulation procedures work in a similar way.

Epidural steroid injections are possibly the most common procedure performed by pain doctors and known by the average person. Their effectiveness and safety has been documented in multiple well-researched studies through the years. An ideal patient would be someone with low back pain that radiates down his or her legs or with upper back pain that radiates to the arms. This pain is usually from pressure on a disc or spinal arthritis on the emerging nerve or spinal column. The procedure involves injection of a mixture of local anesthetic and a long-acting steroid around the offending nerve under X-ray guidance in an operating room setting. Many patients notice some immediate relief from the local anesthetic and weeks of sustained relief from the steroid. The procedures may be repeated as needed. As in other procedures, there is a possibility of complications, but the chances are very low in expert hands.

Many cases of reflex sympathetic dystrophy/complex regional pain syndrome (RSD/CRPS), postherpetic neuralgia (PHN), and other so-called sympathetically maintained pain (SMP) respond to a sympathetic block, although more than one injection may be needed. Patients that respond temporarily to a sympathetic block may benefit from a longer-lasting ablation procedure or a neurolytic procedure. The ablation procedure involves the use of heat from a radio-frequency system, a corrosive agent, or cryogenic systems.

The ablation procedures are also effective for axial upper, lower back pain, chronic knee pain, sacroiliac pain, and some cancer pain, such as from abdominal cancers.

Often we use diagnostic nerve blocks to confirm the origin of a patient's symptoms. That knowledge may then be used to formulate a plan, including a longer-lasting procedure or a surgical option. Patients usually are not sedated before a diagnostic nerve block, although some people with anxiety (or low pain threshold) may need a small amount of medication during the procedure. Even then, patients need to be conscious and responding either to facilitate targeting and/or to reduce the risks of unintended complications.

I hasten to add here that the basic nerve blocks mentioned above then break down into dozens of specific procedures for certain areas of the body. It is not "one procedure fits all" by any means.

Despite the variety of available nerve blocks, they may not be for everyone. In fact, in some patients nerve blocks may be risky and thus contraindicated. The main "absolute" contraindications include patient refusal, infection at the site of the block, and allergies to the intended medications. There are also other so-called relative contraindications. Patients taking blood thinners like coumadin for their heart or another condition need to be carefully managed if a spinal injection is planned. If a block is performed while a patient is on a blood thinner, there is a risk of bleeding that may compress the spinal cord and lead to paralysis of the lower extremities if no urgent surgical decompression procedure is undertaken. Patients should not stop these medications without consulting their physician. In situations like this, I work with the patient's prescribing physician or cardiologist to see if it is safe for the patient to stop this medication for a few days before the procedure. Then a blood test is recommended to confirm a safe profile and a spinal procedure is performed. After the block, the patient can restart the medication. Similar guidelines are adhered to for spinal and other blocks and for newer blood thinners like Plavix, though the time spans for starting and stopping the medications vary.[1]

On the flip side, nerve blocks have obvious advantages over drug treatment, although the two are often employed in tandem. When performed by a trained and experienced practitioner, they can be microtargeted and have low risks. In addition, they result in better patient compliance and offer the benefit of avoiding medications like opioids, with their inherent risks of addiction, drug interactions, and serious side effects such as respiratory depression and death.

Even if the results of some nerve blocks may not be permanent—and few are—giving a patient respite from pain can be beneficial beyond the obvious. Besides easing his or her hurt, this may provide a window of time for the patient to begin (or step up) physical therapy to achieve strength, core building, stamina, and wider range of motion. This, in turn, may have long-lasting effects of its own.

NEUROMODULATION

Another approach to consider is neuromodulation. This a relatively new, revolutionary concept that has undergone major and rapid advances in the last few decades. The North American Neuromodulation Society (NANS) defines *neuromodulation* as "the application of targeted electrical, chemical and biological technologies to the nervous system in order to improve function and quality of life."[2] Types of neuromodulation currently employed include spinal cord stimulation

(SCS), peripheral nerve stimulation (PNS), deep brain and cortical stimulation (DBS), and intrathecal drug delivery systems.

Intrathecal drug delivery systems, or so-called pain pumps, are used for the continuous infusion of pain and other medications directly into the spine through a programmable, implanted pump. Because the delivery is targeted to a specific site, a very small amount of medication is needed, as opposed to if a drug was given by mouth, through the skin, or through other routes. This reduces the risks and side effects of these drugs. However, the pumps need to be refilled at regular intervals, usually monthly, and that requires a visit to the doctor. As with other procedures, there are risks and complications, including accidental overdose.

SCS is a pain-relief technique that continuously delivers a low-voltage electrical current to the spinal cord to block the sensation of pain. SCS is the most commonly used implantable neurostimulation technology for management of pain syndromes. As many as fifty thousand neurostimulators are implanted worldwide every year. SCS is a widely accepted, FDA-approved medical treatment for chronic pain of the trunk and limbs (back, legs, and arms). Specific conditions include the pain resulting from arachnoiditis, complex regional pain syndrome (CRPS), failed back surgery syndrome (FBSS), postlaminectomy syndrome (lumbar or cervical), nerve damage, neuropathy, or neuritis.

There are three SCS device types:

- **Conventional systems** require little effort on the patient's part for maintenance. However, a minor surgical procedure is required to replace the power source when it runs out.
- **Radio-frequency [RF] systems** are designed to sustain therapy over long periods at the highest output level. Because of its high-power capabilities, the RF system is suitable for the most challenging cases in which there is complex, multi-extremity pain. With this type of system, the patient must wear an external power source to activate stimulation.
- **Rechargeable systems** are the newest type of SCS device. The patient is responsible for recharging the power source when it runs low. A rechargeable system typically lasts longer than a conventional system. Eventually a minor surgical procedure may be required to replace the power source if the time between recharges becomes impractical.[3]

The first use of small electrical currents as a human analgesic was reported in 1971—a Japanese team found that by sending small electrical currents through wires running along the epidural space—the outermost part of the spinal canal—they could disrupt the crippling pain signals being sent back to the brain, and replace them with a more acceptable buzzing sensation.[4]

Like anything else, SCS may not always work. From what I've witnessed, though, in some cases it can produce spectacular results. Many of my patients have been through several failed back surgeries and have tried heavy doses of opioids and were told that they would probably never walk again. In some of these cases, the SCS has not only significantly decreased their pain level, but it has reduced the amount of pain medication they need and restored their mobility.

Before putting in a permanent implant, a period of trial, temporary stimulation is attempted. The leads are planted and the device programmed for the patient's specific area of pain. The patient is instructed on the device's use and discharged home for a few days. He or she thus gets to experience the effects in real, everyday situations.

After about a week, and if the device seems to be reducing the symptoms as expected, the procedure is repeated, but this time a pulse generator is also implanted. The incision is relatively small, and the wire goes through the epidural space on top of the spinal cord. Up to sixteen or more electrodes can be attached to the leads, allowing for a multitude of programming and relief to a relatively large area.

According to an article in the *Korean Journal of Pain*:

> The exact mechanisms of pain relief by SCS still remain unknown. The basic scientific background of the SCS trials was based initially on the Gate Control Theory of pain, described by Melzack and Wall. In this theory, they proposed that the stimulation of large non-nociceptive myelinated fibers of the peripheral nerves (A-β fibers) inhibited the activity of small nociceptive projections (A-δ and C) in the dorsal horn of the spinal cord. However, it seems that other mechanisms may play a more significant role in the mechanisms of action of the SCS.[5]

Dr. Richard North, a professor of neurosurgery at Johns Hopkins University School of Medicine is someone who has been one of those at the forefront of using and assessing this technology. In a study, he concludes that "SCS is more effective than reoperation as a treatment for persistent radicular pain after lumbosacral spine surgery, and in the great majority of patients, it obviates the need for reoperation."[6]

Studies looking into the long-term results of SCS have reported generally good results. In one study,

> twenty-one percent of the patients never experienced any pain relief. Of the remaining 80, 75% were still using the stimulator. Fifty-one percent of the 80 patients were experiencing good to excellent results and 20% moderate results. There was no reduction over time in the amount of pain relief in patients who initially had at least 75% pain relief. Patients with initial pain relief between 50% and 74% observed a moderate reduction in their pain relief after two years. Patients who initially experienced less than 50% pain relief observed a dramatic reduction in their results in the long term follow-up.[7]

PERIPHERAL NERVE STIMULATION

A relatively recent approach for the relief of chronic pain is the minimally invasive peripheral nerve stimulation or PNS. The published literature suggests that PNS provides significant results in some patients. In addition, the technique is less invasive and does not require the doctor to go through the epidural space that is needed for SCS, minimizing the serious complications that the latter approach may lead to.

The International Neuromodulation Society (INS) describes PNS as

> a commonly used approach to treat chronic pain. It involves surgery that places a small electrical device (a wire-like electrode) next to one of the peripheral nerves. (These are the nerves that are located beyond the brain or spinal cord.) The electrode delivers rapid electrical pulses that are felt like mild tingles (so-called paresthesias). During the testing period (trial), the electrode is connected to an external device, and if the trial is successful, a small generator gets implanted into the patient's body. Similar to heart pacemakers, electricity is delivered from the generator to the nerve or nerves using one or several electrodes. The patient is able to control stimulation by turning the device on and off and adjusting stimulation parameters as needed.

A common misconception about PNS is that it is a relatively new method that was just recently introduced. In fact, PNS was invented in the mid-1960s, even before the commonly used spinal cord stimulation (SCS). Since that time, PNS has become established for very specific clinical indications, including certain complex regional pain syndromes, pain due to peripheral nerve injuries, etc. Some of the common applications of PNS include treatment of back pain (recently approved in some parts of the world), occipital nerve stimulation for treatment of migraine headaches, and pudendal nerve stimulation that is being investigated for use in urinary bladder incontinence.[8]

The first groundwork for the neuromodulation was set forth by Wall, Street, and Sheldon and continued for twenty years with minimal proficiency and technology.[9] For a variety of indications such as PHN, trigeminal neuropathy/neuralgia, migraines and cluster headaches, trigeminal and occipital nerves have remained major nerves to receive PNS. Other conditions that have been shown to respond to PNS include postsurgical pain, low back pain, scapular pain, coccydynia, and CRPS.[10]

Many of the past device-related adverse events in PNS emerged from its off-label use of conventional SCS equipment. The lengthy leads, the tunneling required for the leads, and the bulky implantable pulse generator (IPG) of the SCS device may not be applicable for the peripheral nerve space, and the complications related to the device could be avoided with other, more suitable device components.[11]

A micro electrode system operated by wireless technology and produced by Stimwave is a major advancement in the field of PNS. Having a novel external wireless power generator (WPG), it uses a "dipole antenna for electric field coupling" achieved with "very short length pulsed electromagnetic waves at Giga Hertz Frequencies (GHz)," also known as microwaves. The smaller implants are capable of being placed successfully by percutaneous minimally invasive techniques.[12]

This miniature system contains four or eight contacts and obtains access by an implantable electrode contact array, a microprocessor receiver, and an antenna coupled to an external WPG. The implant is passive and operated by the WPG in accordance with the patient-physician protocol as needed for therapeutic effects. The wide range of parameters ready for use for stimulation consist of an amplitude, pulse width, and frequency. Placement of the electrodes at the targeted nerve with PNS is proposed to change the blood flow, concentration of local neurotransmitters, and endorphins, as well as cell membrane polarization, thus inhibiting the nociceptive transmission.[13]

With encouraging results, wireless neuromodulation is making the way for an expanding array of indications for pain relief of chronic pain conditions. The uncomplicated placement of the device without the need to tunnel and implant an IPG can be favorable to the patient, surgeon, and the healthcare system by reducing costs, procedure time, postoperative pain, and adverse events while gaining the desired pain control.[14]

All stimulation techniques offer the advantage of long-term relief without the need to follow up with a physician too often. This is a definite plus for patients who are too busy or too weak to follow up frequently.

With new research and advanced tools and techniques, we now have the opportunity and ability to use these advances for some patients suffering from chronic pain and thus reduce, and potentially eliminate, the need for risky medications like opioids.

We have come a long way, but the mission to "perfect the work" and "sharpen our tools," which Confucius referred to in this chapter's epigraph, goes on.

16

ALTERNATIVE MANAGEMENT OPTIONS

When it comes to alternative treatments for chronic pain, I find myself somewhat on the fence.

Having grown up in an Eastern culture, from childhood I became familiar with acupuncture, yoga, tai chi, and other concepts that are only now taking hold in the Western world under the "new age" umbrella. Moreover, I have been told by more than a few chronic pain patients that some of these things have indeed helped to moderate their discomfort.

Certainly, chronic pain is in a category all its own when it comes to connecting the mind and body. Theoretically, at least, if the brain can tell the body that it should feel pain even when there seems to be no physical reason for it, then it seems logical that the process could be reversed. Couldn't the brain be "tricked" somehow into telling the body that something that should hurt really doesn't? This is part of what many of these "new age" modalities purport to address.

Since chronic pain is often exacerbated by depression and stress, most of the alternative approaches to managing that pain involve some form of relaxation therapy. In the case of tai chi and yoga, enticing the body to move (just as in physical therapy) is often helpful, both on a mental and muscular level.

Our charge as physicians is *primum non nocere*, or "first, do no harm." I try to apply that philosophy to alternative chronic pain therapies. I have no problem with a patient using them in conjunction with more traditional methods of healing, as long as there is no potential for making the condition worse. For example, I have become intrigued with, and convinced of, cognitive behavioral therapy (CBT) and biofeedback as possible weapons against pain.

On the other side of the fence, however, is a natural skepticism. Things like acupuncture and chiropractic care are viewed with a certain amount of suspicion by the medical community as a whole because there is limited evidence that they are effective in the long term and/or safe. Most traditionally trained physicians share this skepticism.

In fairness, of course, this same medical community has yet to find a cure for most types of chronic pain or even a standard explanation for why it exists. Even so, we are trained with knowledge to locate, diagnose, and manage that pain; knowledge that is gained in four to five years of medical schooling and an additional three to five years, or more, of a grilling medical residency and fellowship. Many foreign medical graduates have to go through this process two times over— once in our former country and then again in the United States. This is the expertise that a person administering an alternative treatment might not possess.

To a cursory observer, there may be commonality between the nerve blocks I administer and the needles used by an acupuncturist. However, this is where the commonality ends. The former is evidence based and proven science that people have learned to trust and accept.

A quick trip through your favorite Internet search engine will probably result more in confusion than enlightenment. Some of the websites extolling the virtues of acupuncture or massage therapy or chiropractic care may not be trustworthy or reliable. Meanwhile, personal accounts of success or failure from some of these treatments probably may have more to do with the very individualized, natural progression of pain conditions than with the efficiency of the treatment itself. And then there is the placebo effect.

The most reasonable advice would be to listen to anyone who offers to help moderate or manage your chronic pain while remaining wary of those who promise an outright cure. Nevertheless, because this is a book dealing with all aspects of chronic pain, it would be irresponsible of me not to spend a little time on alternative healing practices. Here are a few of the more prominent ones.

ACUPUNCTURE

After hearing about a person's symptoms, and perhaps some personal background, the acupuncturist will decide which points on the body to address. He or she then swabs these places with alcohol and inserts metal needles at different depths. In some cases, electricity or heat may be added.

A paper published by the health and psychology department at Vanderbilt University provides the following rationale for this practice, which dates back more than twenty-five hundred years.

> Qi (pronounced "chee") serves as the life force that circulates throughout the body. It is accumulated, balanced and enhanced by the dietary intake and air. Disorder and sickness are caused by the unbalanced, obstructed and irregular flow of Qi. Meridians are simply channels that carry Qi throughout the body. They are composed of acupuncture points that form a specific pathway. Acupuncture, by stimulating specific acupuncture points, is able to regulate the Yin and Yang and Qi in the body and, therefore, treat the sickness or disorder.
>
> Acupuncture has been claimed effective for various pain conditions including migraines, back pain, tennis elbow, menstrual cramps, fibromyalgia and carpal tunnel syndrome. However, there exist studies that have not found acupuncture an effective approach in treating certain other pains like osteoarthritis. These studies suggest acupuncture as no more effective than placebo. Acupuncture seems to be a safe and effective therapy for certain health problems, but further, more controlled research is needed to establish a firmer ground for the efficacy of acupuncture in treating various chronic pains.[1]

The first impulse of any Western-trained physician is to dismiss all talk of "Qi" as so much mumbo jumbo. Scientifically, there is no link between these "meridians" and the nerve networks carrying pain information to the brain. And the "acupuncture points" do not approximate the location of the nerves themselves. There is no convincing evidence that the needles used in acupuncture result in increasing the endorphins and other natural painkillers.

CHIROPRACTICS

At its heart, this treatment form is hands-on. Quite literally. It involves the physical manipulation of the spine, other joints, and soft tissue.

Spinal manipulation and chiropractic care may be considered relatively safe, but there have been some proven cases of severe damage. In 2016, Playboy model Katie May is reported to have died days after experiencing a stroke caused by a ruptured artery, and it was reported that the artery was damaged during a neck manipulation by a chiropractor.[2] More recently, in September 2017 a U.S. district court in Virginia settled at mediation a case of stroke caused by vertebral artery dissection that occurred after a chiropractic manipulation.[3]

If you have certain conditions like spinal cord compression, inflammatory arthritis, osteoporosis, or are taking blood thinners, it would not be wise to have any spinal manipulations done.

Also, the chiropractor should have a thorough knowledge of your medical history and your current medical conditions and be able and willing to refer you for medical consultation if a serious complication does arise. He or she should be informed of any medications you are taking, high-risk lifestyle factors you may have, and any surgical history. Prior knowledge of a chiropractor's track record is recommended.

The impression from the medical side is that some chiropractors have been unwarranted in expanding their scope of treatment from back and neck pain (and headaches that might have been caused by spinal problems) into virtually the entire range of chronic pain and other medical issues.

Like acupuncture, chiropractics exists as an alternative—or, perhaps, an adjunct—to standard medical treatment. Only a few states (New Mexico was the first) allow chiropractors to prescribe medications, and most states bar them from performing any but the most rudimentary forms of surgery.

The consensus of the medical community, which relies on evidence-based knowledge, would be to disregard any extravagant claims of a permanent cure.

MASSAGE

Like acupuncture, this might be a positive addendum to a more traditional approach. But as with chiropractics, it is best entered with a clear knowledge of the person who will be doing the work.

In an article written for the Practical Pain Management website, Brenda L. Griffith of the American Massage Therapy Association noted:

> The Joint Commission on Accreditation of Healthcare Organizations (JCAHO) suggests massage as a non-pharmacological therapy that can be used successfully in pain management. Some hospitals are including massage therapists in patient care teams to fight pain. Their teams may include a physician, several nurses, a nutritionist, a yoga instructor, a chaplain, and a massage therapist. Often, the hospitals are including massage because of public demand. More research needs to be done to evaluate not only the effectiveness of such teams, but of the various elements within them, to determine which combination of therapies works best for different types of patients and different types of pain. [4]

The problem that practitioners of massage have always encountered, especially in terms of gaining acceptance from the medical profession, is that the term *massage therapist* can cover everything from spa employees to illegal massage parlors. Many states have gone to certification policies to weed out the latter, but the line between *relaxation massage* and *medical massage* (a term that has increasingly come into general use since the mid-1990s) is often indistinct.

In most cases, massage is less intrusive than chiropractic care. Also, massage meshes well with certain types of chronic pain.

Often in neuropathic conditions such as reflex sympathetic dystrophy/complex regional pain syndrome (RSD/CRPS), postherpetic neuralgia (PNH), or fibromyalgia, a muscle's reaction to pain is to spasm, which causes more pain. That pain, in turn, triggers another spasm. Massage can sometimes ease those spasms and help to break that vicious circle.

Medical massage practitioners have made fibromyalgia a special focus, especially since that condition is believed to be rooted in the muscles and joints. It also provides a sort of body road map with its various "trigger points."

Massage gives many people a sense of relaxation and well-being, perhaps because it stimulates serotonin and endorphins. Once again, though, it is a tool for managing and moderating chronic pain, not for ending it.

BIOFEEDBACK AND COGNITIVE BEHAVIORAL THERAPY (CBT)

This also brings me back to my Eastern roots, but in a different way. Mind control over the body is an ancient art practiced by Hindu holy men, allowing them to seemingly ignore what others would deem excruciating pain (lying on a bed of nails while weights are piled upon them, for example).

Biofeedback takes some of the same traditions, packages them for acceptance within a technological Western culture, and helps chronic pain patients help themselves.

> In a biofeedback session, sensors attached to your body are connected to a monitoring device that measures body functions such as breathing, perspiration, skin temperature, blood pressure, and heartbeat. When you relax, clear your mind, and breathe deeply, your breathing slows and your heart rate dips correspondingly. As the numbers change on the monitors, you begin to learn how to consciously control body functions that are normally unconscious. For many patients, it can be a powerful, liberating experience.[5]

Beyond that, according to Rick Thomas, a Kansas City psychologist who uses biofeedback extensively in his practice,

> through a training process, the person is then able to bring his brainwave states under voluntary control. Therefore, he can increase the under-aroused brain or slow the over-aroused brain. This has been shown clinically to affect the chronic pain condition. It is like any other learning process. By giving appropriate feedback, the individual is able to gradually gain control over his psychological and physiological functioning. The more EEG biofeedback training a person undergoes, the more mastery he gains.[6]

The website LifeMatters.com provides a little background as to how a person might arrive at the office of someone like Thomas:

> Symptoms of physiological tension might not be noticed immediately when you encounter stress, and if the response is unnoticed, it can form into a dysfunctional habit, gradually, over time. For example, bruxing or clenching your teeth is normal under stress. However, if the stressor persists the bruxing/clenching habit can "take on a life of its own" so that when the initial stress subsides the bruxing/clenching continues, creating long term problems after the initial stressor has been withdrawn.
>
> In another way, chronic habits that previously were not a problem can become painful. For example, if you are involved in an accident and injure a muscle, the muscle tissue becomes more sensitive. If high levels of tension were previously present and unnoticed, they now contribute to the pain. This often happens with chronic neck and shoulder tension.
>
> For example, a habit develops outside of your awareness, becomes chronic and eventually leads to TMJ problems. In another example, chronic unconscious tension which was not a source of pain before an accident becomes an aggravating factor to injured tissue. In both these examples the tension is outside of your awareness, but the pain isn't. You don't realize the source of the pain and don't know how to alter the muscle tension in order to help reduce the pain or you may not be aware that tension can aggravate pain.[7]

The drawback to this particular modality is that it isn't for everyone. As with the art of meditation, biofeedback requires a degree of concentration of which some people are simply not capable. It is also most effective with body functions (or malfunctions) that directly involve tension, such as blood pressure, muscle spasms, and irritable bowel syndrome.

Still, what I like about biofeedback is that, like physical therapy, it gives the patient the feeling of actively confronting his or her pain and attempting to defeat it. Activity is always preferable to passivity.

The *Free Dictionary* defines *cognitive behavioral therapy* as "an action-oriented form of psychosocial therapy that assumes that maladaptive, or faulty, thinking patterns cause maladaptive behavior and 'negative' emotions (Maladaptive behavior is a behavior that is counterproductive or interferes with every-day living.) The treatment focusses on changing individuals thoughts (cognitive patterns) in order to change his or her behavior and emotional state."[8]

A report in *American Psychologist* discusses the role of CBT as follows:

> CBT is the "gold standard" psychological treatment for individuals with a wide range of pain problems. The efficacy of CBT for reducing pain, distress, pain interference with activities, and disability has been established in systematic reviews and meta-analyses. Although average effect sizes are small to moderate across pain outcomes, CBT lacks the risks associated with chronic pain medications, surgeries, and interventional procedures. Furthermore, CBT may well have benefits for common comorbid conditions such as diabetes and cardiovascular disease. Research is needed to develop CBT interventions that have stronger beneficial effects, with attention to whether tailoring therapy to specific patient subgroups or problems enhances outcomes. Increased understanding of the most effective ingredients of CBT for specific subgroups is integral to treatment improvement and patient–treatment matching. Unfortunately, most individuals with chronic pain never receive CBT. Integration of CBT into medical settings where individuals with chronic pain are commonly seen, especially primary care settings, offers much promise in both expanding application of CBT and improving outcomes, but such approaches are only beginning to be studied.[9]

Approaches like biofeedback and CBT are often effective for chronic pain as part of a comprehensive management plan that may include physical therapy, targeted interventional procedures, and medications. Most other CAM (complementary alternative medicine) treatments may or may not help, and some may result in serious complications. It is prudent that chronic pain patients seek the advice of a medical practitioner before embarking on any approaches that may be potentially harmful.

17

MARIJUANA—THE MYSTERY DRUG

We, as pain doctors, are sometimes confronted with a situation where either the patient informs us that they have been taking marijuana for pain relief or they test positive for this drug during a random urine drug screen while under a pain management contract. Well-informed and well-experienced physicians would offer differing opinions on what to do in this situation.

As discussed elsewhere, most pain practices require patients to sign a pain management contract with their providers at the start of their treatment. Some may only require this if they plan to prescribe opioids. If the patients are prescribed opioids, as a part of that contract, they agree to comply with the recommendations about dosage and frequency of medications prescribed and not take medications or substances that are not prescribed by the physician. The patients are regularly monitored and routinely and randomly screened for compliance. Patients who fail are taken off their opioid pain medications, switched to nonopioid regimens, and may be referred for management of substance abuse disorder.

The confusion in the scenario described above ensues because not all experts agree that marijuana is a "dangerous drug." In addition, many experts believe that it is also less likely that this medication in isolation would result in serious health issues or fatality.

Marijuana—also called *weed, herb, pot, grass, bud, ganja, Mary Jane,* and a vast number of other slang terms—is a greenish-gray mixture of the dried flowers of *Cannabis sativa.* Some people smoke marijuana in hand-rolled cigarettes called *joints*; in pipes, water pipes (sometimes called *bongs*), or in *blunts* (marijuana rolled in cigar wraps). Marijuana can also be used to brew tea and, particularly when it is sold or consumed for medicinal purposes, is frequently mixed into foods (*edibles*) such as brownies, cookies, or candies. Vaporizers are also increasingly used to consume marijuana. Stronger forms of marijuana include sinsemilla (from specially tended female plants) and concentrated resins containing high doses of marijuana's active ingredients, including honeylike *hash oil*, waxy *budder*, and hard amberlike *shatter*. These resins are increasingly popular among those who use them both recreationally and medically.

The main *psychoactive* (mind-altering) chemical in marijuana, responsible for most of the intoxicating effects that people seek, is *delta-9-tetrahydrocannabinol* (THC). The chemical is found in resin produced by the leaves and buds primarily of the female cannabis plant. The plant also contains more than 500 other chemicals, including more than 100 compounds that are chemically related to THC, called *cannabinoids*.[1]

In more general terms, there has been a major discussion on the health, financial, and social effects of marijuana use in the general population. Those in favor cite data that suggests that legalizing this substance has more potential benefits than risks.

The American Civil Liberties Union published a paper called *The War on Marijuana in Black and White*. It concludes as follows:

> Like America's larger War on Drugs, America's War on Marijuana has been a failure. The aggressive enforcement of marijuana possession laws needlessly ensnares hundreds of thousands of people in the criminal justice system, crowds our jails, is carried out in a racially biased manner, wastes millions of taxpayers' dollars and has not reduced marijuana use or availability. Marijuana possession arrests also waste precious police resources and divert law enforcement from responding to and solving serious crimes. It is time for marijuana possession arrests to end.[2]

According to a report by the National Institute on Drug Abuse, marijuana has both short- and long-term effects on the brain. The short-term effects start in thirty minutes to an hour and result in the typical "high" that people feel. These include altered senses, sense of time, mood changes, difficulty thinking, or impaired memory. Especially when people begin using marijuana at a younger age, it may result in thinking, memory, and learning dysfunction. These effects may be permanent. The physical effects may also include breathing problems, increased heart rate, and problems with child development during and after pregnancy. Long-term use may also lead to hallucinations, paranoia, and worsening schizophrenia.[3]

There has been major political and social movement toward legalizing marijuana. Medical marijuana is broadly legalized in twenty-nine states and legalized for recreational use in many others.

A report on *Politico* discusses this further:

> California was the first state to legalize medical marijuana in 1996, largely in response to the AIDS crisis. Over the next decade, other western states followed suit. Then during the Obama administration, medical marijuana spread to every corner and every region of the country, including Washington, D.C., Guam and Puerto Rico. Like other culture war issues such as gay marriage, marijuana found favor with the general population, seemingly overnight after decades of work. In 2012, Colorado citizens voted to become the first state to legalize weed for purely recreational purposes, leaving the federal government in a bit of a pickle. Marijuana was still considered by the feds to be more dangerous than cocaine, so what was it going to do about the eruption of grow operations? One solution would have been to reclassify marijuana out of Schedule I—the list of drugs like heroin considered the most dangerous and addictive and which are deemed to lack any medicinal value—but that didn't happen because of entrenched opposition from the Drug Enforcement Administration and an apparent lack of will at the White House to go to war with its own DEA. Instead, the DOJ wrote a memo as a short-term work-around, drafted by a deputy attorney general named James Cole. Published in August 2013, the four-page Cole Memo was addressed to all U.S. attorneys and said, "In jurisdictions that have enacted laws legalizing marijuana in some form . . . conduct in compliance with those laws and regulations is less likely to threaten the federal priorities. . . ." Translation: Don't go out of your way to prosecute marijuana cases. It was a half-hearted solution that had the effect of giving states some breathing room, but marijuana activists knew that it was just a memo, lacking the force of law.[4]

In December 2018, Attorney General Jeff Sessions reversed the protections offered by the Cole Memo, opening the options for the federal government to prosecute anyone found in possession of marijuana in states where the drug is legal on a state level.

A working paper report by David Powell, Rosalie Liccardo Pacula, and Mireille Jacobson published by the RAND Corporation concludes that states providing legal access to marijuana through dispensaries experienced lower treatment admissions for addiction to pain medications. It also provides complementary evidence that dispensary provisions also reduce deaths due to opioid overdose. They estimate even larger effects in states that have both legally protected and active dispensaries.[5]

Despite wide acceptance nationwide, marijuana is still considered a Schedule I drug by the Drug Enforcement Agency (DEA), along with LSD, heroin, and ecstasy. This identifies them as substances with no currently accepted medical use and a high potential for abuse. Other commonly prescribed opioids like methadone, oxycodone, and morphine are in Schedule II drugs. These are defined as drugs with a high potential for abuse, with use potentially leading to severe psychological or physical dependence. Then there are stepwise Schedules III through V with sequentially lower potential for abuse. Benzodiazepines like Xanax, Ativan, and Ambien are in Schedule IV.

Opioid pain medications and substances like heroin kill thousands of people every year. In contrast, marijuana appears far less toxic, and the deaths related to this substance seem to be mostly related to its effects on decision making, thereby resulting in accidental deaths.

The fight for the legalization of marijuana is ongoing, and in coming years many more states are expected to either legalize it partially for medical use or open it up for recreational use.

Those who favor opening up marijuana use cite statistics of its low social impact, as described above. Those who oppose legalization highlight the point that marijuana may be a "gateway drug" that leads to addiction to other potentially more harmful substances.

At this point, the jury is still out. Many social, political, and economical factors are at play and will decide the final outcome regarding the greater accessibility of this drug.

18

PAIN IN THE COURTROOM

Those who do not feel pain seldom think that it is felt.

—Samuel Johnson

Law and medicine have always been intertwined, but that prickly relationship becomes even more complicated in the area of chronic pain.

More than most other specialists, pain doctors need to keep one eye on recent advances in medicine and the other on how these changes are playing out in legislation and courtrooms.

For while most medical transactions are nonadversarial (barring the occasional malpractice suit), physicians dealing in chronic pain often find themselves embroiled in two very different areas of controversy—government drug policies and financial claims by chronic pain patients.

The former can place the doctor on the ragged edge between legal and illegal activity. The latter can result in a lot of time spent testifying in insurance and workman's compensation cases.

In "Pain Disorder, Hysteria or Somatization?" Harold Merksey neatly combined these two dilemmas: "Pain used to be a simple issue," Merksey wrote. "It was caused by physical injury or disease, and the sufferer had to rest and take opium. That was about two hundred years ago."[1]

Now what used to be strictly medical has become infused with collective morality (the drug issue) and money. As Michael Finch points out in "Law and the Problem of Pain," printed in the *University of Cincinnati Law Review*:

More than ten percent of the population—predominately women—
suffer from chronic pain, and it is often incurable. The resulting
personal and social costs are great. Approximately $85 billion to $100
billion are spent annually for the diagnosis and management of
chronic pain. Almost half of the Social Security disputes pending in
federal court involve claims of chronic pain. Damages for "pain and
suffering" are often the largest component of personal injury awards,
and the perennial focus of tort reform.

Despite the prevalence of chronic pain, one question will not go
away: Is the pain medically "real"? Pain is a quintessentially subjective symptom and no practicable tests exist to verify or quantify its
presence.[2]

That's where the pain specialist enters the picture, often in a scenario where all we can offer from the witness stand is educated speculation. True, in cases of chronic pain from an old injury, we can refer to
MRIs or other objective tools that will demonstrate good reason for the
patient's discomfort. In many cases, however, the body's pain-reporting
system seems to have gone haywire, sounding a shrill alarm with no
threat in sight.

And that's assuming the complainant is not doing it for personal
reasons, hoping to turn pain into gain.

"I wear my crown of thorns upon my liar's chair,"[3] Johnny Cash sang
late in his career—but in the courtroom, that thorny headpiece is all too
often invisible.

It has been my experience that the vast majority of my patients come
to me with an honest evaluation of their medical problem and a legitimate need for relief. And while there are some shysters and malingerers
and scheming personal injury lawyers out there—I'm not naive—the
fact that the people I treat are mostly referred by other physicians
throws up another layer of insulation from bogus complaints.

I do make it a practice to try to observe some patients when they
don't know they're being watched. If their gait, body language, and the
manner in which they get in and out of a chair are different than when
I'm in the room with them, it raises a red flag with me.

Certainly, chronic pain can be lucrative. In his book *Why We Hurt:
The Natural History of Pain*, Dr. Frank Vertosick noted:

During the original Inquisition, pain was used by authority figures as a tool to extract something of value from victims—a confession, money, an oath of loyalty, the betrayal of a friend. But the situation has been turned on its head. Today, some may use pain to leverage something of value from authority figures, usually insurance companies or the government.[4]

As a rule, my testimony in personal injury and workman's compensation cases is anything but dramatic. Here is what the tests said, this is what the patient said to me, this is what I observed. I recall one case in which I wasn't even sure which side my testifying was helping, because, as usual, I was sticking to the facts and the truth.

Yet while I am not a lawyer (my brother took that route), it's easy to see that courts at all levels are still sorting through the concept of chronic pain. In one sense, the evolution of decisions has roughly paralleled a growing acceptance of the idea that pain can exist with no obvious, provable cause. This change has not occurred in a straight line, however, and there are hundreds of occasions in which more conservative judges and juries have rejected chronic pain claims altogether.

It wasn't until 1987, for example, that an Illinois case became the first to use the term *fibromyalgia* instead of *chronic fatigue syndrome* in a decision.[5]

Two years before this, however, a Canadian court decision opened a legal door for fibromyalgia sufferers, at least in that country. As attorney Richard Hayles explained in his presentation "Defending Chronic Pain and Chronic Pain Claims," the trial judge in *Eddie v. Unum Life Insurance Company* noted:

> The fundamental misconception of the defense is that it is necessary to be able to identify the cause of a condition, before benefits under the insurance policy are triggered. One can recognize that insurers may be more comfortable when they have objective evidence of disease. But it is the fact of sickness, not its explanation, which must govern.
>
> I conclude that the meaning of "sickness" in this disability insurance policy includes the condition of a person who genuinely wants to continue in his or her employment but, because of a perception, based on symptoms, that something is wrong with his or her body, genuinely and reasonably feels unable to do so. This is a substantially subjective test and depends on the credibility of the claimant.[6]

Although Canada, like the United States, also produced verdicts that were more hostile to claimants, Hayles describes a general trend toward redefining the employee-employer relationship where chronic pain was concerned.

> In order to be considered disabled, the insured must establish that his pain keeps him from working to the standard of a reasonable employer. If the insured's past employment has normally been full-time, this means that he will be considered disabled if he lacks the capacity to work a full day on a regular basis. Judges do not expect that the insured will be able to find an employer who can accommodate his need for flexible hours, frequent breaks, a specially designed workspace and equipment and other variations in the normal conditions of full-time employment, in the absence of evidence that such an employer actually exists.[7]

Yet the law, like everything else, is constantly pushed and swayed by new advantages in technology—medically or otherwise. Today, unlike the early 1980s, it is possible for a white-collar employee to work at home via computer, and that has sometimes been found to be a solution for both parties.

The tendency of most people in the community of chronic pain sufferers is to sometimes cast insurance companies and employers as the villains in legal proceedings. Nevertheless, there are certainly reasonable expectations on both sides, and the murkiness of chronic pain can allow either side to potentially cross the line and take advantage of the other.

"When the plaintiff claims to be suffering from a chronic condition that has completely altered his life and prevents him from working," writes Hayles, "the court will expect that he has sought medical treatment, and will want to know what his physicians say about his condition, treatment and prognosis."[8]

Yet unanswered questions lurk in virtually every chronic pain case. Take, for example, a plaintiff with chronic back pain suing his former employer for requiring him to lift heavy objects.

Is the pain real? How can this be determined when there are no overt signs of injury? If it is real, is it truly as severe as the plaintiff claims? And even if it's real, and severe, what proof is there that it was caused by the heavy lifting and not some previous injury?

The term *psychosomatic* used to be synonymous with *imaginary*. And since women are more prone than men to conditions such as fibro-myalgia, a certain residual sexism often rears its head in contentions that female pain had "hysterical" origins.

Lawyers arguing against paying damage claims have also blamed stress, depression, or mental illness for unproven pain. In his *Cincinnati Law Review* article, Michael Finch talks about the "chicken or the egg" aspect of this reasoning.

"Clinicians frequently observe a great deal of psychological distress in chronic pain patients," he wrote. "This distress can be interpreted as the source of medically unexplained pain. However, the diagnosis over-looks the fact that chronic medical illness often causes a significant amount of psychological disturbance."[9]

The question, then, becomes: Is the patient in pain because she's depressed or depressed because she's in pain? Studies have been con-ducted on various groups of patients with similar chronic pain to deter-mine whether there was a higher level of stress, previous psychological trauma, or mental illness within that sample. Invariably, the incidence of those factors is no higher than that exhibited by a random sample of the general population.

However, even now, gaining disability benefits is often a struggle for chronic pain sufferers. One of my patients, a woman with the triple whammy of fibromyalgia, arthritis, and lupus, was turned down several times on the basis of those afflictions.

"They finally gave me disability, but not for any of that," she told me. "I got it for IBS [irritable bowel syndrome]."

According to the Americans with Disabilities Act, "A person has a disability if he/she has a physical or mental limitation that substantially limits one or more major life activities, a record of such impairment, or is regarded as having such an impairment."[10]

Certainly, chronic pain almost always fits the first requirement. The next two, however, can be highly subjective. Is a "record of such impair-ment" merely a statement that someone came to a health professional with a chronic pain complaint, or is it an indication that the presence of chronic pain was likely from a medical standpoint? If item 2 is not satisfied, item 3 becomes moot.

Kenneth Mitchell, a physician and vice president of the Chattanoo-ga-based Return to Work Program, notes:

The health and disability insurance industry's reliance on evidence-based medicine requires clear, tangible and objective pieces of information to treat and determine the degree of work incapacity.

Ambiguity, subjectivity and invisibility invite a disability insurance paradox. This paradox states: "Anyone who invests great amounts of time and energy having to prove they cannot work, will not work." Unfortunately, this is the essence of chronic pain management and the subsequent determination of work capacity. [11]

Sometimes, rest areas are offered along the road to disability, especially for employees who are perceived as valuable. But it can be too little, too late.

The good news is, at least some of the suspicion once brought to bear on chronic pain cases by the Social Security Administration (SSA) has been washed away by the avalanche of anecdotal evidence. A paragraph contained in the SSA's five-step process explains:

The Social Security Administration is required to evaluate the intensity, persistence and functionally limited effects of the pain, i.e., how does this pain affect the individual's ability to do basic work activities. Because symptoms, such as pain, sometimes suggest a greater severity of impairment than can be shown by objective medical evidence alone, the adjudicator is required to carefully consider the individual's statements about his/her pain with the rest of the relevant evidence in the case record. An individual's statement about the intensity or persistence of pain or about the effect the pain has on his/her ability to work may not be disregarded solely because they are not substantiated by objective medical evidence. [12]

The flip side is that claimants must be sensitive to the natural skepticism of governmental agencies like SSA. After all, not every crown of thorns is real. Con artists do exist.

The Social Security Disability Resource Center lists a few factors that might sway the opinion of disability adjudicants and workman's compensation judges:

1. You must describe your pain with accuracy and with specificity. Avoid comments like "I hurt all over and I am in constant pain." Instead, describe each part of your body that hurts and what the pain feels like.

2. Chronic pain often results in a level of depression. If you suffer with chronic pain, Social Security judges will expect that you will seek mental health counseling and/or pain management. If there is no evidence of counselling or pain management in the record, many judges will conclude that your pain really is not all that bad.

3. Many people use allegations of chronic pain to convince their doctors to prescribe powerful narcotic pain medications. Judges are very sensitive to this problem. A red flag for judges is an individual who receives pain medication from two or more doctors who are not aware of one another.[13]

And what about insurance companies? Here, the sticking point may be the nature of chronic pain rather than its actual existence. Since chronic pain often doesn't go away, insurers find themselves staring uncomfortably down a long road lined with company-issued checks.

Will Rowe, CEO of the American Pain Foundation, explained, "With pain, usually it's a multi-modal form of treatment that works best."[14]

But many insurance companies, like many doctors, are solution oriented. They want quick fixes and often suggest surgery as an early option in hopes of solving the problem. Some are open to alternative therapies such as acupuncture, massage, and yoga; others are wary. Still others will pick and choose their way through the "multimodal" strategy as if it were a salad bar.

"They might not cover the physical therapy," said Rowe, "but they'll cover the medicine. Or, if they cover the physical therapy, they only cover three sessions."[15]

Rowe also recommends making sure your doctor is on your side and not taking an initial denial from the insurance company as the definitive answer.

"Find out your insurance company's procedures for appealing a denial and follow up," he advises.[16]

No matter how much it hurts to do so.

As Robert Frost would say, "The best way out is always through."

19

COEXISTING WITH PAIN

That which does not kill us makes us stronger.

—Friedrich Nietzsche

Or to paraphrase that gloomy German philosopher just a bit: That which does not kill us must be dealt with.

Although chronic pain does make some people stronger, others collapse under its weight. Living with it instead of struggling against it generally means hard work and slow progress, and it requires commitment.

Therefore, while I would never tell a patient, "This is always going to hurt, so accept it and stop complaining," nor would I promise to rid the patient of his or her discomfort completely and forever.

Those of us who wage war on chronic pain know that there is seldom a full-scale retreat by our enemy. Instead, we operate somewhere between victory and defeat, hoping for a solution that allows our patients to function as normally as possible.

As is the case with life in general, managing chronic pain involves understanding and accepting reasonable expectations.

A few years back, I had a female patient who went from doctor to doctor and received multiple medications without relief. More than the pain itself, she was more frustrated that no one seemed to understand what her symptoms were resulting from. She had fatigue, difficulty sleeping, and difficulty indulging in even minimal everyday activities. After a thorough evaluation and excluding other possible conditions, we figured out that she was suffering from fibromyalgia. Incidentally, she had not been given this diagnosis for the previous few years that she was being managed for pain. I explained to her that this is a condition that may be life-long, but with lifestyle changes, including aerobic exercise programs and targeted medications like duloxetene and/or pregrablin, and possibly trigger-point injections as needed, we may be able to keep the symptoms under control. We have achieved that goal, but more significantly she is more relieved that she knows what her diagnosis and prognosis is. She is comfortable with her situation.

This is not to say that chronic pain is never curable. Sometimes it really does go away, maybe even as the result of a correct diagnosis and effective treatment by the physician. Other times, the doctor might be as mystified as anyone else as to why that happy accident occurred.

In his book *Why We Hurt: The Natural History of Pain*, Dr. Frank T. Vertosick Jr. writes:

> Some neurophysiologists believe that chronic pain resides in the brain, not the body. Although the original source of the pain might be outside the brain—as ruptured disc or broken bone—this bodily pain can eventually activate a pain center in the brain, perhaps in the thalamus, and once activated, it's never silent again. Quite literally, the problem is "all in our heads."[1]

This is both good and bad news for chronic pain sufferers. While it seems more logical to attend to pain at what appears to be its source, the brain has proven itself quite welcoming to pain-relieving chemicals and impulse modulation. It even produces its own, the magical endorphins.

But that's not the kind of brain power this chapter is about. As with any other battle, defeating—or at least neutralizing—chronic pain requires a strategy. And a strategy requires thought. Furthermore, there is no template, because everyone's pain journey is unique. Only you know how much it hurts and how often it hurts. You know what the pain allows you to do and which doors it has closed to you.

Learn the movements of your enemy. It is helpful to keep a diary of your pain, listing when it peaks and wanes and how it feels as the day unfolds. Over time, if you're lucky, patterns will emerge. For example, a person with rheumatoid arthritis might experience the worst pain in the morning, before the afflicted joints have loosened some with movement. With fibromyalgia, fatigue may join the pain late in the afternoon.

Once you know how your pain behaves, you can perhaps work around it to some degree. It's a bit like the weather. If you live in a hot climate and it's summertime, it's probably best to stay inside during the hours the sun is at its highest point. You can't negotiate with the sun to accommodate your schedule, and chronic pain is often just as intractable.

One of the many downsides to experiencing chronic pain, then, is a certain loss of spontaneity. Activities often must be arranged to work around your discomfort. If you're having a bad day, it would obviously be unwise to attack a superhuman schedule of work. (Note: Be wary of trying to do too much on a good day, either, because the following morning could be three steps backward.)

It may also be instructive to keep track of how you are feeling emotionally. It's no secret that depression feeds on pain the way sharks are attracted to blood. Try to maintain your perspective during down periods—if you're feeling sad or angry or hopeless for no specific reason, it probably has more to do with fatigue or pain than the fact that your neighbor didn't wave at you when you walked to the mailbox. If the pain is keeping you from restorative sleep at night, try taking a nap during the day. As football coach Vince Lombardi once said, "Fatigue makes cowards of us all."

The Mayo Clinic on Chronic Pain, edited by Dr. Charles Swanson, offers a useful acronym in terms of goals: SMART (specific, measurable, attainable, realistic, trackable). Take the future in small bites. If you allow yourself to consider the possibility of enduring the same discomfort for ten or fifteen years, paralysis of will may set in. Try to avoid thinking about that and embrace that old cliché: "One day at a time."[2]

Another oft-repeated phrase might also serve as a helpful mantra: "Give me the patience to accept the things I cannot change, the courage to change what I can change, and the wisdom to know the difference." This humble prayer takes on added complexity with chronic pain, however. What may be changeable one day must be accepted the next.

Knowledge of one's condition is a key element in dealing with pain. It's almost a certainty that if a person were to be told that his or her pain stems from an incurable, probably terminal illness, it would hurt more than if the discomfort was attached to something less grim.

Having worked in an emergency room, I can tell you that the outward appearance of an injury—or the pain associated with it—does not necessarily coincide with severity. In his book, Frank Vertosick Jr. relates the case of a man who was brought into an ER by ambulance after (he said) almost amputating his thumb. He had immediately wrapped a cloth around the thumb after the accident and kept it there during his trip to the hospital, complaining of extreme pain. But when the cloth was removed, it turned out to be just a small cut, and the patient immediately felt his pain diminish.[3]

Or as physicians Chris Wells and Graham Nown, along with Ronald Melzack, write in *The Pain Relief Handbook*, part of the power of knowledge is

> realizing that the severity of pain is not related to the severity of illness. Anyone can die just as easily from a painless heart attack as from a painful one.
>
> Some forms of cancers, particularly the leukemias, can be quite malignant without being painful at all. Other types of cancers are extremely painful, but this has no bearing on the severity.[4]

Realizing this takes fear out of the equation. Nietzsche never heard of fibromyalgia or reflex sympathetic dystrophy (RSD), but he did suffer from painful arthritis much of his life and knew that it wouldn't kill him—even though there were probably days when he hoped it would.

Again, Wells, Nown, and Melazack state:

> Your attitude toward pain should not be that it is something enormous and terrible because you have suffered for so long. By changing your perspective and rationalizing what you feel, you can tell yourself "If the pain has been there for that length of time, perhaps I don't need to take so much notice of it."[5]

Perhaps my greatest frustration as a pain specialist is when I run up against patient passivity. Part of this, I realize, is the fault of medical history. Until fairly recently, we took our pain to bed on "doctor's orders" and left the doctor's office clutching a slip of paper excusing us from work or school.

"You'd better stay off that for a while," we were told.

Sometimes, naturally, that's good advice. No one should be hobbling around on a badly broken leg or torn ligament. In most cases, though, exercise will not worsen chronic pain. And if the pain comes from a ruptured disc or other form of injury, a physical therapist can suggest exercises that will not aggravate the condition but help improve them.

Physical therapy is, in fact, the ideal place for chronic pain patients to start a workout program, and I almost write more prescriptions for that than I do for pain-killing drugs.

If you suffer from chronic pain, you may have spent a lengthy sedentary period convalescing, or you may worry that exercise might cause you further damage. The physical therapist can deal with both of those concerns, and you'll find that exercising on a regular basis—with help and advice—will get you past the time when it is difficult to get started.

Exercise has a number of benefits for anyone dealing with chronic pain:

1. A general deterioration in physical condition is often a parallel problem for chronic pain sufferers. The more they hurt, the less they do. Soon, the weight piles on, the muscles become stiff, and a descending spiral is set in motion. Only a regular regimen of exercise will pull the patient out of this decline.
2. Exercise, when done vigorously, can stimulate the body's production of endorphins—the proverbial "runner's high."
3. Exercise relieves tension and stress.
4. Working out can provide a distraction from thinking about the pain.
5. Exercise provides a sense of becoming a part of one's own treatment. Rather than simply relying on his or her doctor and prescribed medications, both of which are somewhat passive solutions, the patient has the satisfaction of offering physical resistance to what is plaguing him or her.

Of course, common sense must come into play. Generally, "low-impact" exercise is the best path rather than weight lifting or marathon running. If the knees, spine, or other joints have been invaded by chronic pain, swimming and water exercises are wonderful ways to strengthen muscles while not putting any more pressure on weight-bearing areas. Cycling and walking are also considered low-risk activities.

Spirituality and religion can be very powerful weapons to fight the feeling of worthlessness and depression that usually accompany misfortunes like chronic illness. When you focus your mind and seek inner guidance, the doors can open and the light can shine again. We have all seen or heard about people with supposedly hopeless conditions who awoke their spiritual selves, broke their shackles, and transformed once again into confident individuals. Individuals at peace with themselves and with the situations around them.

Mindfulness and yoga is another possibility. Writing for the Website Inner Idea, yoga therapist Robin Rothenberg has these suggestions for chronic pain patients who feel drawn to a mind-body activity for relief:

> Start with relaxed breathing in a supported position, such as lying down. Break down complicated classical yoga poses into simple movements and stretches. Individuals with chronic pain may hold tension in many areas of the body, and have many pain triggers. Use props, such as blankets or chairs, to make poses more accessible. [6]

In any form of exercise, listen to your body. It will tell you quite bluntly if you have crossed the line. Where you seek relief may depend on your personality. A naturally high-energy individual who feels constrained and suppressed by chronic pain might choose an activity that will pump up the heart rate. A more meditative type might choose, well, meditation. And there are always safer, nonopioid antipain drugs to enlist in the fight, if we use them wisely.

It's important to realize that these antipain medications are meant to be an ally, not a crutch.

Their function is to help us with our pain, not to provide intoxication and entertainment. Distraction from pain does not mean creating yet another problem—that of addiction—to be confronted.

True, there are times when pain can be hell. Or as one of the characters in Jean-Paul Sartre's play *No Exit* famously observed: "Hell is other people."

For a chronic pain sufferer, this is often true. Most of us don't hurt in a vacuum—we have spouses, children, friends, parents, bosses, co-workers, and a host of other people who care about us and are thus affected by our pain and how we choose to handle it. In the process, they sometimes trigger feelings of guilt and irritation that drag us down even more.

It's hard suffering from chronic pain, but it's also hard when someone close to you is in that situation. This is something to think about when we are asked the inevitable question: "How are you today?" Often the honest answer is "terrible." Unfortunately, this response puts the questioner in an awkward position. Does this person sympathize with you? Is sympathy what you really want?

A guide to chronic pain published by the Mayo Clinic puts it well:

> People around you generally react in one of two ways to pain behaviors. They become annoyed by them—"Not this again"—or they become overly attentive to the behaviors—"Here, let me do that." Either response creates an unequal relationship in which people tend to focus more on your behavior than on your thoughts or feelings.[7]

Interacting with others despite chronic pain is like exercising under the same circumstances—difficult but necessary. What you don't want to do is become a prisoner at home. Instead of always requesting visitors to come to you, try to get out to lunch or dinner and meet with the people in your life in a different setting. Answer any questions about your condition honestly, and wait for them to bring the subject up.

Most people, especially close friends, will understand. If you continually rebuff their attempts to get together with you, however, they may eventually decide you would rather be left alone. To counter that, reach out with phone calls and e-mails to let them know they are still on your mind. Ask about their lives, and try to keep any venting about your own problems to a minimum.

Relations with family members can be more difficult. They are more directly affected, and a bout of chronic pain can wreak havoc on the structure of a household. Suddenly, the person who usually prepares the meals has trouble cooking. There is no one to mow the grass. A prolonged, pain-driven absence from work shrinks the family income dramatically. Beyond that, someone in pain is not always easy to live with. That person may become increasingly prickly because of his or her discomfort and the unwanted changes that condition has made in his or her daily routine. Despite all efforts at understanding, that occasionally wears thin.

As always in any relationship, frank communication is paramount. Something like "I'm really sorry I snapped at you. My back is really bothering me today, and it's put me in kind of a bad mood" will go a long way to smooth things over. But if it's not always advisable to complain to friends or family, where should the outlet be? Like a kettle on the stove, a person in chronic pain has to occasionally let off steam. It's also difficult to make other people understand what you're going through when it is something they have never experienced.

This is where a support group might be helpful. They exist for almost every affliction known to man, and if there isn't one in your community that deals with your particular problem, chances are you can find it online.

A woman named Susan L. Gardner, writing on the blog *ZebraMichelle*, posted "The 12 Steps of Living with Chronic Pain." It is, I believe, worth repeating here:

1. I am powerless over chronic pain and it makes my life unmanageable. I do what I can and the rest will have to wait until I get to it.
2. I refuse to feel guilty about having a health condition that limits but does not stop my life. Chronic pain guilt will eat you up. Let it go. . . . Make the best of what you have and live.
3. I will do a fearless inventory on my losses and my emotions. I will explore my past, relationships with my family, friends, co-workers, and employers. In an effort to gain perspective of how chronic pain has affected my past; and, in order to be at peace with my present, and gain hope for the future.
4. I am willing to make amends where necessary. I'm sure along the way I have made others angry, and for that I am sorry. However, I refuse to take on any un-necessary responsibility or guilt that does not belong to me.
5. I refuse to accept mislabeling in my life. I will no longer accept terms like lazy, crazy, mental, addicted, malingering, seeking secondary gain, hypochondriac or any other of the countless, thoughtless titles included in the stigma of chronic pain to be allowed in my life. I am a human being as well.
6. I will remember to pace myself. Take things one step at a time in my recovery process. I am not out of the race, I just have to run a little slower.

7. I am willing to take responsibility for my illness by use of research and advocacy in order to make the best decision for ME. After all, I am the one living this life.

8. I refuse to accept that I can no longer be a viable person and believe that my God has, in his infinite wisdom, a purpose designed, just for me.

9. I will seek out a healthy balance of life. These include medical, spiritual, emotional, social, psychological and physical health. In addition, I will seek out joy, peace, love and laughter.

10. I know that chronic pain affects every aspect of my life; but, does not have to control my life. I must learn to look at life in a different light by finding new ways to do old things.

11. I will remember that living with chronic pain affects my family, as well as myself. And, in order to stay a healthy family, we must learn to communicate.

12. Most importantly, I want to share my journey, showing care, warmth, respect, encouragement and understanding to my chronic comrades in life.[8]

All good advice, for the medical profession can only go so far. There are no more Marcus Welbys who will come to your house and discuss your prognosis over tea—if that person ever existed in the first place. Your time with someone like me is short, and you then have to take your problem home and live with it. It's hard, but it can be done.

And ultimately, no one else can do it for you.

20

TOWARD A PAIN-FREE FUTURE

The medical community has come a long way over the past fifteen years in the fight against chronic pain.

The first step in this fight, however, was identifying chronic pain as a worthy foe.

Historically, many doctors would rarely ask their new patients if they were in pain—a question any parent would pose to their child immediately after a fall. The emphasis of treatment was on finding the root of the problem and solving it. It was just simply assumed that pain would be present until the problem was solved.

These physicians weren't being neglectful or cruel. If a patient complained of pain, he or she would be prescribed some sort of pain reliever. Physicians were just not trained to treat pain as a separate force to be reckoned with. This means that in cases where no visible cause of pain was evident, relief was even harder to find.

What came out of a Chicago conference of the Joint Commission on Accreditation of Healthcare Organizations (JCAHO) in May 2000 was, in a very real sense, an emancipation proclamation for people suffering from afflictions such as reflex sympathetic dystrophy/chronic regional pain syndrome (RSD/CRPS) or fibromyalgia.

In a paper on these standards, Patricia Berry and June Dahl report:

> The newly approved Joint Commission on Accreditation of Health-care Organizations (JCAHO) pain management standards present an important opportunity for widespread and sustainable improvement in pain assessment and management. Unrelieved pain is a major, yet

avoidable, public health problem. Despite 20 years of work by educators, clinicians, and professional organizations and the publication of clinical practice guidelines, there have been, at best, modest improvements in pain management practices. Multiple barriers found in the health care system, and among health care professionals, patients, and families, continue to impede progress. In August 1997 a collaborative project was initiated to integrate pain assessment and management into the standards, intent statements, and examples of implementation of JCAHO—a rare opportunity to improve pain management in health care facilities throughout the country. After review by multiple JCAHO committees and advisory groups and critique by an expert panel, the JCAHO Board of Commissioners approved the revisions in May 1999. The revisions are published in the 2000–2001 standards manuals and will be effective January 1, 2001, for all patient care organizations accredited by JCAHO—ambulatory care, behavioral health, health care networks, home care, hospitals, long-term care, and long-term care pharmacies.[1]

Founded in 1951, The Joint Commission accredits and certifies more than 21,000 health care organizations and programs in the United States. An independent, nonprofit organization, The Joint Commission is the nation's oldest and largest standards-setting and accrediting body in health care. To earn and maintain The Joint Commission's Gold Seal of Approval®, an organization undergoes an on-site survey by a Joint Commission survey team at least every three years.[2]

In other words, JCAHO had serious clout, and pressure from groups such as the American Pain Society convinced its members that pain needed to be looked at in a different way. A new set of standards was drawn up in 1999, with the goal of making pain "a fifth vital sign."[3]

It wasn't until the spring conference a year later, though, that these new JCAHO standards were disseminated beyond the boardrooms and medical schools to the general public. As a young doctor just entering the pain field, I felt validated and encouraged by all of this, especially the requirement for better education. I knew that it would only help me if family practitioners, nurses, and other people in the medical field became more knowledgeable.

In order to pass the standards, medical providers were required to

- Screen for the existence and assess the nature and intensity of pain in all patients.
- Recognize the right of patients to appropriate assessment and management of pain.
- Record the results of the assessment in a way that facilitates regular reassessment and follow-up.
- Determine and ensure staff competency in pain assessment and management, and address pain assessment and management in the orientation of all new staff.
- Establish policies and procedures that support the appropriate prescription or ordering of effective pain medications.
- Educate patients and their families about effective pain management.
- Address patient needs for symptom management in the discharge planning process.
- Maintain a pain control performance improvement plan.[4]

Seeing pain as an enemy in and of itself was only the first step, of course. Once the pain was recognized and dealt with, its cause had to be identified. Once identified, the cause had to be treated. And once treated, at least in a perfect world, the condition needed to be cured.

There are many institutes working on pain research: the National Institutes of Health, the National Institute of Neurological Disorders, the National Institute of Dental and Craniofacial Research, the National Cancer Institute, the National Institute of Nursing Research, the National Institute on Drug Abuse, and the National Institute of Mental Health. The primary goal of pain research is, of course, to develop better pain treatments.

One of the best things about the medical field is that there are, in general, no secrets. It's hard to imagine a doctor coming up with a special drug or technique to more effectively deal with chronic pain and then keeping it to him- or herself. Such innovations are almost always reported in medical journals, presented at conferences, or revealed in some other public fashion.

Like politics and the stock market, medical research is driven by numbers. Rare diseases that afflict relatively few people generally sink to the bottom of the list for research grants. The major pharmaceutical companies that often fund medical research want to see drugs that will help large masses of people—and, by extension, sell millions of pills. That's not necessarily a bad thing, just the way the economy works.

The National Institutes of Health (NIH) in an analysis in 2015 "found that an estimated 25.3 million adults (11.2 percent) experience chronic pain—that is, they had pain every day for the preceding 3 months. Nearly 40 million adults (17.6 percent) experience severe levels of pain. Those with severe pain are also likely to have worse health status."[5]

The more chronic pain takes center stage, then—and it's been featured on both *Time* and *Newsweek* covers in recent years, as well as on every major news network—the more researchers gravitate toward solving the unique problems it presents.

At this point, the focus is more on treatment than cure. Just as the crews scrambling to plug the 2010 oil leak in the Gulf of Mexico weren't as concerned about how the accident happened as how to stop it, so pain doctors have learned to deal with the symptoms even when they're stumped for a cause.

Short of a cure, though, we all crave a quicker route to diagnosis. Often time is critical with a chronic pain case. The longer a "let's try this and see if it works, then try something else if it doesn't" approach is taken, the more intractable the condition can become.

Part of the solution is greater cooperation between family physicians, emergency room doctors, and other primary care providers and those who specialize in chronic pain. I've noticed, from my perspective, that these physicians are quicker to call a pain doctor for a referral—or just a consultation—than they used to be.

So what have we learned about chronic pain since I came into the field more than a decade and a half ago, fresh from the University of Virginia?

American Pain Foundation president Scott Fishman says:

> We know exponentially more today than we knew even 10 years ago and much more than we knew 50 years ago. For one, we've learned a great deal about how pain is produced and transmitted and perceived. Fifty years ago, when someone hurt, we thought it was just a symptom of something else. But we now know the symptom of pain can become a disease in and of itself, and that disease is similar to other chronic conditions that can damage all aspects of someone's life.

For all we've learned, however, we have not translated most of these advances to the frontline of medicine. Every time we take one of these discoveries and treat accordingly, we find unwanted side effects because pain is so pervasive. For instance, it's very hard to give someone pain relief without making them sleepy. It's very hard to turn off the nerves that transmit pain without producing the risk of seizure or heart rhythm problems. But we're making advances. We're learning more about the electrical channels involved in nerve function. And we have many more candidates to target, and we're very hopeful that's going to translate into drugs with far fewer side effects.[6]

One of the beneficial side effects of chronic pain research in recent years has been to bring two seemingly diverse groups of specialists—pain doctors and mental health practitioners—closer together as allies. The merger has even resulted in a new hybrid, the pain psychologist. One of this new breed, Philadelphia-based David Kannerstein, summarizes the emerging paradigm:

One of the most important areas where people with chronic pain can benefit from psychological help is in changing negative thoughts and beliefs which help prevent more effective coping. These thoughts and beliefs can also worsen the pain and suffering the person with pain experiences by reinforcing and deepening negative emotional states including anxiety, depression, and anger. Examples of negative thoughts related to pain would be "I am useless," "I am worthless," "I can't do anything to control this pain," "no one believes I am in this much pain," etc. In turn, these thoughts reflect underlying beliefs such as "I'm only valuable as a person if I am working," "I am no good if I have to depend on others for help," and so on. In our society, which emphasizes financial gain, work productivity, and individual autonomy, these are very common beliefs. However, while they may be functional to a point by inspiring us to work hard and achieve what we can, they become serious liabilities if we become disabled.[7]

In short, the dismissive "It's all in your head" has given way to "Let us into your head, so we can help." We now understand that the brain can be a coconspirator in creating chronic pain, both in interior thoughts and physical dysfunction.

This insight has given rise to new technology such as functional magnetic resonance imaging (fMRI) and positron emission tomography (PET), both of which use injected dyes to track the movement and activity of blood vessels in the brain. This movement can indicate whether or not a person is in pain and even how much. Research has also shown that chronic pain inhabits some of the same areas of the brain as certain emotions.

On one hand, such information can be helpful. On the other hand, it only emphasizes the individuality that makes chronic pain so difficult to treat. A medication that works well for one species of chronic pain may not help at all with another variation. Even within the parameters of the same condition, there can be major differences in treatment approaches from one individual to another.

As much as I enjoy solving a medical mystery, it would make my job infinitely easier if I could test a chronic pain patient, arrive at a clear-cut diagnosis, then use the same treatment I used yesterday on someone else with the same condition.

Some conditions discussed elsewhere in this book, such as postherpetic neuralgia (PHN), RSD/CRPS, and even fibromyalgia, are becoming more clear-cut as time and research progress. Others, including chronic headaches and certain types of back pain, remain maddeningly elusive. When also considering the aforementioned mental and emotional components, coming up with a one-size-fits-all treatment for any type of chronic pain is still a way off.

In October 2011, for example, ABC's nightly news program featured a Texas woman named Linda Brown who had been suffering from a condition known as trigeminal neuralgia. Since 2002, Brown said, she had been experiencing facial pain so severe and unremitting "that I ceased to be able to exist."[8]

Her agony was no mystery. It was caused by a pain-transmitting nerve in her brain being squeezed by two blood vessels. Neurosurgeon Dong Kim at the University of Texas Hospital went in, cushioned the nerve with a tiny piece of felt, and the pain immediately stopped.

"He is my miracle man," Brown said.[9]

Would that work for other chronic pain patients with conditions such as RSD/CRPS? Probably not, because Linda Brown's situation was rare. That much-trumpeted surgical intervention did, however, illustrate the current trend toward being more proactive with chronic pain.

I trust the efficiency of and remain committed to minimally invasive procedures for many patients with chronic pain. These may be a nerve block, an ablation procedure, or a peripheral nerve or spinal cord stimulation to ease discomfort, both in the short and long term. Sometimes, however, surgery—sometimes major surgery—such as to relieve the pressure on a spinal nerve or spinal cord, becomes essential to regain the function. In case of back pain, this is particularly true if an emergency situation when limb weakness or bladder or bowel dysfunction is present.

Opioids, although potent and effective medications, on the other hand, are fast losing their past luster because of the safety issues as the devastating opioid crisis looms large.

Fortunately, there is groundbreaking research underway to develop innovative medications swiftly and safely for many ailments, including chronic pain.

In December 2016, President Barack Obama signed into law the 21st Century Cures Act, which "builds on FDA's ongoing efforts to advance medical product innovation and ensure that patients get access to treatments as quickly as possible, with continued assurance from high quality evidence that they are safe and effective."[10]

In June last year, Pfizer and Lilly "announced that U.S. Food and Drug Administration (FDA) granted Fast Track designation for tanezumab for the treatment of chronic pain in patients with osteoarthritis (OA) and chronic low back pain (CLBP). Tanezumab is an investigational humanized monoclonal antibody that selectively targets, binds to and inhibits nerve growth factor (NGF)."[11]

We know that our body has its own endogenous opioids like endorphins, enkephalins, dynorphins, endomorphins, and nociceptins. These, and other exogenous medications like narcotics medications, work on opioid receptors. By their effect on these receptors, they result in not only pain relief or analgesia but other serious and unwanted side effects, including physical dependence, addiction, anxiety, euphoria, constipation, sedation, and respiratory depression. Many cases of opioid-related fatality are related to severe respiratory depression.

New medications are being developed to microtarget a subset of these receptors that may result in analgesia without other undesired effects. In addition, other medications are in the pipeline that may act on receptors other than the opioid receptors that may be involved in pain generation or transmission. These include calcium channel, transient receptor potential of the vanilloid type (TRPV), and N-methyl-D-aspartate (NMDA receptors).

A new paper points to the fact that drug research has so focused on "trying to prevent the propagation of action potentials in the periphery from reaching the brain rather than pinpointing . . . the receptor itself." They discuss the newly identified nociceptive receptors that have changed this rationale. Transient receptor potential (TRP) channels are involved in "mechanical, chemical and thermal stimuli detection." This has become a viable drug target for clinical use in the management of pain.[12]

Oxytocin is known to the medical profession as a hormone that is released by the posterior pituitary in response to the stretching of the uterus and cervix and facilitates childbirth. It is also released on stimulation of the nipples, which helps breastfeeding and bonding.

Beneficial effects of oxytocin have been noted in studies of anxiety, depression, sexual dysfunction, and drug addiction. Taken together, oxytocin also appears to have potential benefits for treating the comorbidities that accompany deep tissue pains and may even treat some of the problems produced by more traditional treatments for pain such as opioids.[13]

Major research is being done on calcitonin gene-related peptide (CGRP), a chemical found in the peripheral and central nervous system and the cerebrovascular system that is believed to be implicated in many conditions, including chronic migraines. "During spontaneous migraine attacks, CGRP concentrations measured from the external jugular vein rise. CGRP serum levels decrease after administration of triptans in parallel with symptomatic relief."[14] In an article in the *New England Journal of Medicine*, the researchers tested erenumab, "a fully human monoclonal antibody that inhibits the calcitonin gene–related peptide receptor, for the prevention of episodic migraine."[15] The clinical data concluded that "erenumab administered subcutaneously at a monthly dose of 70 mg or 140 mg significantly reduced migraine frequency, the effects of migraines on daily activities, and the use of acute migraine–specific medication over a period of 6 months."[16] The research funded by Amgen and Novartis is poised to place Aimovig, a novel, targeted option in the hands of clinicians to help patients suffering from this debilitating chronic pain condition.

And those are just a few of the innovative therapies, out of many others, that are being aggressively researched. Add to that the massive, ongoing research to understand the complex conditions that result in so much suffering.

In a sense, as pain doctors we are contributing to put ourselves out of business. One by one, specific chronic pain conditions are being moved from the "mystery" pile to the realm of standard treatment.

Someday, perhaps, that process will be completed. And I will be a happy person, for I would see at least some of the misery wiped off the face of those I care for most.

NOTES

INTRODUCTION: A LONG WAY
FROM KASHMIR

1. Abdul Majid Zargar, "Mahatma Gandhi and Kashmir Politics," *Greater Kashmir*, November 2, 2011, www.greaterkashmir.com/news/gk-magazine/mahatma-gandhi-and-kashmir-politics/105106.html.

I. MEDICATIONS THAT RELIEVE PAIN—AND KILL

1. T. Christian Miller and Jeff Gerth, "Behind the Numbers," ProPublica, September 20, 2013, www.propublica.org/article/tylenol-mcneil-fda-behind-the-numbers.

2. Gurkirpal Singh, "Recent Considerations in Nonsteroidal Anti-inflammatory Drug Gastropathy," *American Journal of Medicine* 105, no. 1 (July 27, 1998): 31S-38S, doi:10.1016/s0002-9343(98)00072-2.

3. "WHO's Cancer Pain Ladder for Adults," World Health Organization, accessed January 12, 2018, www.who.int/cancer/palliative/painladder/en/.

4. "Overdose Death Rates," National Institute on Drug Abuse, revised September 2017, www.drugabuse.gov/related-topics/trends-statistics/overdose-death-rates.

5. Celine Gounder, "Who Is Responsible for the Pain-Pill Epidemic?" *New Yorker*, June 19, 2017, www.newyorker.com/business/currency/who-is-responsible-for-the-pain-pill-epidemic.

6. Ibid.

7. Scott Fishman, quoted in mem6526, "Addiction vs. Dependence," MDJunction, accessed January 8, 2018, www.mdjunction.com/forums/panic-attacks-discussions/general-support/3688958-addiction-vs-dependence.

8. Marion S. Greene and R. Andrew Chambers, "Pseudoaddiction: Fact or Fiction? An Investigation of the Medical Literature," *PMC: US National Library of Medicine National Institutes of Health*, October 2015, accessed January 8, 2018, www.ncbi.nlm.nih.gov/pmc/articles/PMC4628053/.

2. THE OPIOID EPIDEMIC THAT IS KILLING US

1. "Terrorism: Death Toll Worldwide 2006–2016," Statista: The Statistics Portal, released July 2017, www.statista.com/statistics/202871/number-of-fatalities-by-terrorist-attacks-worldwide/.

2. "Overdose Death Rates," National Institute on Drug Abuse, revised September 2017, www.drugabuse.gov/related-topics/trends-statistics/overdose-death-rates.

3. Steven Ross Johnson, "Trump Declares the Opioid Crisis a Public Health Emergency but Won't Dedicate More Money to Fight," *Modern Healthcare*, October 26, 2017, www.modernhealthcare.com/article/20171026/NEWS/171029906.

4. Centers for Disease Control and Prevention, *Annual Surveillance Report of Drug Related Risks and Outcomes—United States, 2017: Surveillance Special Report 1* (Atlanta, GA: Centers for Disease Control and Prevention, U.S. Department of Health and Human Services, August 31, 2017), www.cdc.gov/drugoverdose/pdf/pubs/2017-cdc-drug-surveillance-report.pdf.

5. Christopher Ingraham, "Where Opiates Killed the Most People in 2015," *Washington Post*, December 13, 2016, www.washingtonpost.com/news/wonk/wp/2016/12/13/where-opiates-killed-the-most-people-in-2015/?utm_term=.e1750fd3cb9e.

6. Josh Katz, "The First Count of Fentanyl Deaths in 2016: Up 540% in Three Years," *New York Times*, September 2, 2017, www.nytimes.com/interactive/2017/09/02/upshot/fentanyl-drug-overdose-deaths.html.

7. "Fentanyl," Opioid Overdose, Centers for Disease Control and Prevention, last updated August 29, 2017, www.cdc.gov/drugoverdose/opioids/fentanyl.html.

8. Ibid.

9. *America's State of Mind*, Medco, 2010, http://apps.who.int/medicinedocs/documents/s19032en/s19032en.pdf.

10.   M. Olfson, M. King, and M. Schoenbaum, "Benzodiazepine Use in the United States," *JAMA Psychiatry* 72, no. 2 (February 2015), abstract, www.ncbi.nlm.nih.gov/pubmed/25517224.

11.   D. Dowell, T. M. Haegerich, and R. Chou, *CDC Guideline for Prescribing Opioids for Chronic Pain—United States, 2016*, MMWR Recomm. Rep. 2016; 65, no. RR-1 (Atlanta, GA: Centers for Disease Control and Prevention, 2016), 1–49, www.cdc.gov/mmwr/volumes/65/rr/rr6501e1.htm.

12.   Ibid.

3. ON ADDICTION MANAGEMENT

1.   American Society of Addiction Medicine (ASAM), *The ASAM National Practice Guideline for the Use of Medications in the Treatment of Addiction Involving Opioid Use*. (Chevy Chase, MD: American Society of Addiction Medicine, June 1, 2015), www.asam.org/docs/default-source/practice-support/guidelines-and-consensus-docs/asam-national-practice-guideline-supplement.pdf.

2.   "Opioid Addiction: 2016 Facts & Figures," American Society of Addiction Medicine, www.asam.org/docs/default-source/advocacy/opioid-addiction-disease-facts-figures.pdf. See also National Institute on Drug Abuse, "Drug Facts: Heroin," National Institute on Drug Abuse website, revised January 2018, www.drugabuse.gov/publications/drugfacts/heroin.

3.   "Opioid Addiction." See also Rob Stein, "Life Expectancy in U.S. Drops for First Time in Decades, Report Finds," NPR, December 8, 2016, www.npr.org/sections/health-shots/2016/12/08/504667607/life-expectancy-in-u-s-drops-for-first-time-in-decades-report-finds.

4.   Blue Cross Blue Shield (BCBS) and Blue Health Intelligence (BHI), *America's Opioid Epidemic and Its Effect on the Nation's Commercially-Insured Population*, Health of America Report (Chicago: Blue Cross Blue Shield, June 29, 2017), 2, accessed January 14, 2018, www.bcbs.com/the-health-of-america/reports/americas-opioid-epidemic-and-its-effect-on-the-nations-commercially-insured.

5.   Ibid. See also R. A. Rudd, P. Seth, F. David, and L. Scholl, *Increases in Drug and Opioid-Involved Overdose Deaths—United States, 2010–2015*, Morbidity and Mortality Weekly Report, December 16, 2016 (Atlanta, GA: Centers for Disease Control and Prevention, 2016).

6.   BCBS and BHI, *America's Opioid Epidemic*.

7.   U.S. Department of Health and Human Services, Office of the Surgeon General, *Facing Addiction in America: The Surgeon General's Report on Alcohol, Drugs, and Health* (Washington, DC: U.S. Department of Health and

Human Services, 2016), chap. 4, https://addiction.surgeongeneral.gov/chapter-4-treatment.pdf.

8. Celine Gounder, "Who Is Responsible for the Pain-Pill Epidemic?" *New Yorker*, June 19, 2017, www.newyorker.com/business/currency/who-is-responsible-for-the-pain-pill-epidemic.

9. National Institute on Drug Abuse, "How Effective Is Drug Addiction Treatment?" in *Principles of Drug Addiction Treatment: A Research-Based Guide*, 3rd ed. (Bethesda, MD: National Institute on Drug Abuse, December 2012), last updated January 2018, www.drugabuse.gov/publications/principles-drug-addiction-treatment-research-based-guide-third-edition/frequently-asked-questions/how-effective-drug-addiction-treatment.

10. Ibid.

11. Quoted in Trung Nguyen, *Naturalopy Precept 14: Wisdom* (N.p.: En-Cognitive, 2015), 3.

4. THE MYSTERY OF PAIN

1. Melanie Thernstrom, *The Pain Chronicles* (New York: Farrar, Strauss & Giroux, 2010): 30.

2. Kenneth L. Casey, "Problems in the Differential Diagnosis of Chronic Pain," *Anesthesia Progress* 37 (1990): 61.

3. Ibid., 63.

4. Karen Uhlenhuth, "The Pain Is Real, but Is Fibromyalgia a Condition?" *Kansas City Star*, March 31, 2003, www.prohealth.com/library/the-pain-is-real-but-is-fibromyalgia-a-condition-depends-on-who-you-ask-21093.

5. Matthew Perrone, "Questionable Disease Boosted by Eli Lilly & Fizer," Associated Press, February 9, 2009, www.cbsnews.com/news/fibromyalgia-disease-or-marketing-ploy.

6. Alex Berenson, "Drug Approved: Is Disease Real?" *New York Times*, January 14, 2008, www.nytimes.com/2008/01/14/health/14pain.html.

7. Alice Sebold, "Reviews of *The Pain Chronicles*," 2010, http://melanie-thernstrom.com/painreviews.html.

5. THE COMPLEX NATURE OF CHRONIC PAIN

1. Dan Simmons, *The Fall of Hyperion* (Grand Haven, MI: Brilliance Audio, 2009), chap. 32.

2. Richard W. Hanson, "The Biological Aspects of Pain," in *Self-Management of Chronic Pain: Patient Handbook* (Wanganui, NZ: Arachnoiditis Sufferers Action & Monitoring Society, 2006), 30.

3. Melanie Thernstrom, *The Pain Chronicles* (New York: Farrar, Strauss & Giroux, 2010), 44.

4. Howard L. Fields, "Pain Perception—the Dana Guide," Dana Foundation, November 2007, www.thblack.com/links/RSD/Pain%20Perception_TheDanaGuide5pp.pdf.

5. Center for Workforce Studies, *2014 Physician Specialty Data Handbook* (Washington, DC: Association of American Medical Colleges, November 2014), www.aamc.org/download/473260/data/2014physicianspecialtydata-book.pdf.

6. THE CULTURE OF PAIN

1. Nick Williams, "Arab Version of Machismo Plays Elusive Role in Mideast Showdown," *Los Angeles Times*, August 28, 1990, http://articles.latimes.com/1990-08-28/news/mn-214_1_arab-public-opinion.

2. Sarah Whitman, "Pain and Suffering as Viewed by the Hindu Religion," *Journal of Pain* 8, no. 8: 609, doi:10.1016/j.jpain.2007.02.430.

3. Ibid., 610.

4. Darlene Cohen, "Mindfulness and Pain," *Darlene Cohen* (blog), 2010. www.darlenecohen.net/welcome/mindfulness.html.

5. Alcira Molina-Ali, dir., *In Search of a Muslim Pain Principle*, video (Houston: Medium, 2004), www.youtube.com/watch?v=7aNcG-GeUl8&feature=youtu.be.

6. Elsa Martinez, "Pain and Race/Ethnicity" (paper for the National Pain Foundation).

7. Ibid.

8. K. E. Lasch, "Culture and Pain," *Pain: Clinical Updates* 10, no. 5 (2002): 8.

9. Gregory I. Elmer, Jeanne O. Pieper, Stevens S. Negus, and James H. Woods, "Genetic Variance in Nociception and Its Relationship to the Potency of Morphine-Induced Analgesia in Thermal and Chemical Tests," *Pain* 75, no. 1 (1998): abstract, doi:10.1016/s0304-3959(97)00215-7.

10. H. Kim, "Genetic Influence on Variability in Human Acute Experimental Pain Sensitivity Associated with Gender, Ethnicity and Psychological Temperament," *Pain* 109, no. 3 (June 2004): abstract, doi:10.1016/s0304-3959(04)00119-8.

11.   Inna E. Tchivileva, Pei Feng Lim, Shad B. Smith, Gary D. Slade, Luda Diatchenko, Samuel A. Mclean, and William Maixner, "Effect of Catechol-O-Methyltransferase Polymorphism on Response to Propranolol Therapy in Chronic Musculoskeletal Pain: A Randomized, Double-Blind, Placebo-Controlled, Crossover Pilot Study," *Pharmacogenetics and Genomics*, April 2010, 1, doi:10.1097/fpc.0b013e328337f9ab.

12.   David Weissman, Deb Gordon, and Shiva Bidar-Sielaff, "Cultural Aspects of Pain Management," *Journal of Palliative Medicine* 7, no. 5: 715, doi:10.1089/jpm.2004.7.715.

13.   Ibid.

7. THE STIGMA OF PAIN

1.   Laura Shocker, "More than Just a Headache: Battling Migraine Stigma," *Huffington Post*, May 16, 2011, www.huffingtonpost.com/2011/05/16/migraine-stigma_n_862255.html.

2.   Ibid.

3.   Ibid.

4.   Ibid.

5.   Marcia Bedard, "Bankruptcies of the Heart: Secondary Losses from Disabling," *Lyme Times* (Chico, CA), Fall/ Winter 2002/3, http://lymediseaseresourcec.bizland.com/archives/LT34.PDF.

6.   Ibid.

7.   Ibid.

8.   Ibid.

9.   Jean Jackson, "Stigma, Liminality and Change," *American Ethnologist* 32, no. 3 (2005): 332.

10. *People* staff, "Paula's Secret Struggle," *People* magazine, May 2, 2005, http://people.com/archive/cover-story-paulas-secret-struggle-vol-63-no-17.

11. Ibid.

12. Bedard, "Bankruptcies of the Heart."

8. SAD BUT TRUE—CHRONIC PAIN AND DEPRESSION

1.   Raven/Missy, "30 Years of Chronic Pain," *Living with Chronic Pain and Depression* (blog), May 6, 2011, https://ravenpain.blogspot.com/2011/05/30-years-of-chronic-pain.html.

2. Kathleen Crowley, "Managing Depression: While Chronic Pain and Depression Can Go Hand in Hand, They Don't Have To," *Lifeline*, Winter 1996, https://walkforhealing.weebly.com/managing-chronic-pain-and-depression.html.

3. Robert J. Gatchel, Yuan Bo Peng, Madelon L. Peters, Perry N. Fuchs, and Dennis C. Turk, "The Biophysical Approach to Chronic Pain: Scientific Advances and Future Directions," *Physiological Bulletin* 133, no.4 (2007): 600, doi:10.1037/0033-2909.133.4.581.

4. Ibid.

5. Harvard Medical School, "Depression and Pain," Harvard Health Publishing, last modified March 21, 2017, www.health.harvard.edu/mind-and-mood/depression-and-pain.

6. Steven Stanos, "Pain and Depression: Pathology, Prevalence, & Treatment," *CNS News Special Edition*, 2005, 35–36.

7. Rollin Gallagher, "The Relationship between Pain, Depression and Mood: An Interview with Rollin Gallagher, MD, MPH," National Pain Foundation, June 4, 2008, www.nationalpainfoundation.org/MyTreatment/News_PainAndDepression_GallagherInterview.asp.

8. Mayo Clinic Staff, "Antidepressants: Another weapon against chronic pain," Mayo Clinic. https://www.mayoclinic.org/pain-medications/art-20045647.

9. Henry J. McQuay and R. Andrew Moore, "Antidepressants and Chronic Pain," *BMJ: British Medical Journal* 314, no. 7083 (1997): 763, doi:10.1136.314.7083.763.

9. OBESITY AND CHRONIC PAIN

1. E. Amy Janke, Allison Collins, and Andrea T. Kozak, "Overview of the Relationship between Pain and Obesity: What Do We Know? Where Do We Go Next?" *Journal of Rehabilitation Research and Development* 44, no. 2 (2007): 245–62, doi:10.1682/jrrd.2006.06.0060.

2. Ibid.

3. "Obesity and Overweight: Fact Sheet," World Health Organization, October 2017, accessed December 27, 2017, www.who.int/mediacentre/factsheets/fs311/en/.

4. Akiko Okifuji, and Bradford Hare, "The Association between Chronic Pain and Obesity," *Journal of Pain Research* 8 (2015): 399, doi:10.2147/jpr.s55598.

5. Ibid. See also Holli A. Devon, Mariann R. Piano, Anne G. Rosenfeld, and Debra A. Hoppensteadt, "The Association of Pain with Protein Inflamma-

tory Biomarkers," *Nursing* Research 63, no. 1 (2014): 51–62, doi:10.1097/
nnr.0000000000000013; Laura-Isabel Arranz, Magda Rafecas, and Cayetano
Alegre, "Effects of Obesity on Function and Quality of Life in Chronic Pain
Conditions," *Current Rheumatology Reports* 16, no. 1 (2013), 390,
doi:10.1007/s11926-013-0390-7.

6. Angela P. Makris and Gary D. Foster, "Dietary Approaches to Obesity
and the Metabolic Syndrome," *Psychiatric Clinics of North America*, 34, no. 4
(December 2011): 813, doi:10.1016/j.psc.2011.08.004..

7. Barbara L. Loevinger, Daniel Muller, Carmen Alonso, and Christopher
L. Coe, "Metabolic Syndrome in Women with Chronic Pain," *Metabolism* 56,
no. 1 (January 2007): 87–93, doi:10.1016/j.metabol.2006.09.001.

8. "Obesity Rates & Trends Overview," State of Obesity, 2016, https://
stateofobesity.org/obesity-rates-trends-overview/.

9. Ibid.

10. Jun Hozumi, Masahiko Sumitani, Yoshitaka Matsubayashi, Hiroaki Abe,
Yasushi Oshima, Hirotaka Chikuda, Katsushi Takeshita, and Yoshitsugu Yama-
da, "Relationship between Neuropathic Pain and Obesity," *Pain Research and
Management*, March 29, 2016, https://www.hindawi.com/journals/prm/2016/
2487924/.

11. Ibid. See also M. E. Bigal, R. B. Lipton, P. R. Holland, and P. J.
Goadsby, "Obesity, Migraine, and Chronic Migraine: Possible Mechanisms of
Interaction," *Neurology* 68, no. 21 (2007): 1851–861, doi:10.1212/
01.wnl.0000262045.11646.b1; Judith J. Wurtman, "Depression and Weight
Gain: The Serotonin Connection," *Journal of Affective Disorders* 29, no. 2–3
(October–November 1993): 183–92, www.sciencedirect.com/science/article/
pii/016503279390032F; A. A. Miller and S. J. Spencer, "Obesity and Neuroin-
flammation: A Pathway to Cognitive Impairment," *Brain, Behavior, and Im-
munity* 42 (November 2014): 10–21, www.sciencedirect.com/science/article/
pii/S0889159114000889.

10. FINDING THE RIGHT SPECIALIST

1. John Loeser, "Leading Figure Describes Current State of Pain Management," ChronicPainDoctor.net, accessed December 2009,
www.chronicpaindoctor.net/.

2. Ibid.

3. Henry Adams, "Chronic Pain Treatment at Camp Pendleton? Observa-
tions of a Credentialed Pain Specialist," ChronicPainDoctor.net, accessed December 2009, www.chronicpaindoctor.net/?cash-loans-online-no-fax.

4. Anthony Kirkpatrick, "Reflex Sympathetic Dystrophy: RSD/CRPS Treatment Center and Research Institute," RSDHealthcare.org, last modified May 2003, www.rsdhealthcare.org/.

5. Bill McCarberg, "Improving the Care of Patients with Chronic Pain: Individualized Assessment and Mechanism-Based Multimodal Treatment" (paper presented at Anaheim Convention Center, Anaheim, CA, May 1, 2013), www.pri-med.com/DigitalAssets/Shared%20Files/Sylla-bus%20Files%20Spring%202013/C&E/West/Track%202-Session%201_Pain_Updates-West_ONLINE.pdf.

6. Scott Mowbray, "Pain Expert B. Eliot Cole, MD, Explains Why Patients Have to Fight for Good Care," *Health* online, last modified March 16, 2016, www.health.com/health/condition-article/0,,20236455,00.html.

7. Chuck Weber, "How Specialists Can Help You Tackle Your Chronic Pain," *Health* online, last modified February 29, 2016, www.health.com/health/condition-article/0,,20188114,00.html.

11. SEARCHING FOR THE CAUSE OF PAIN

1. Cleveland Clinic Foundation, "What Pain-Prone Disorder Is and What It Has to Do with Depression?" *Know Depression from the Inside Out* (blog), last modified 2011, https://knowdepression.wordpress.com/what-pain-prone-disorder-is-and-what-it-has-to-do-with-depression/.

12. FIBROMYALGIA *BECOMES* REAL

1. Melanie Thernstrom, *The Pain Chronicles* (New York: Farrar, Strauss & Giroux, 2010),141.

2. Ivanhoe Broadcast News, "Validating Fibromyalgia: Behind the Pain," interview with Daniel Clauw, MDJunction, www.mdjunction.com/forums/fibro-and-chronic-fatigue-discussions/medicine-treatments/10637038-validating-fibromyalgia-behind-the-pain.

3. Cassie Osborne, "My Life with Fibromyalgia," *Cassie's Site* (blog), 1999, www.clho.net/per/fibro.php.

4. Julie Wendell, quoted on ADiseaseADay.com (site discontinued).

5. Ibid.

6. Terry S., "Who Is Fibromyalgia?" Fibromyalgia-Treatment.com, accessed January 6, 2018, http://fibromyalgia.techie.org/fibromyalgia-demographics/.

7.   "Does Fibromyalgia Run in the Family," Fibromyalgia-Symptoms.org, accessed January 6, 2018, www.fibromyalgia-ymptoms.org/fibromyal-gia_genetics.html.

8.   "The Great Gift of Legitimacy," Fibromyalgia-Symptoms.org, accessed January 6, 2018, www.fibromyalgia-symptoms.org/great-gift-of-legitima-cy.html.

9.   Ibid.

10.   Gina Shaw, "Fibromyalgia: Is Fibromyalgia Real?" *Neurology Now* 5, no. 5 (2009): 29, doi:10.1097/01.NNN.0000361358.53768.86.

11.   Ibid., 30.

12.   "Fibromyalgia Tender Points and Trigger Points," WebMD, accessed August 13, 2011, www.webmd.com/fibromyalgia/guide/fibromyalgia-tender-points-trigger-points#1.

13. OTHER PAIN CONDITIONS

1.   Florian T. Nickel, Frank Seifert, Stefan Lanz, and Christian Maihöfner, "Mechanisms of Neuropathic Pain," *European Neuropsychopharmacology* 22, no. 2 (2012): 81–91, doi:10.1016/j.euroneuro.2011.05.005.

2.   Keith Orsini, quoted in "What Is CRPS? What Is RSD?" American RSDHope, 2017, accessed January 6, 2018, www.rsdhope.org/what-is-crps1.html.

3.   Nickel et al., "Mechanisms of Neuropathic Pain."

4.   Anthony F. Kirkpatrick, ed., *Reflex Sympathetic Dystrophy Clinical Practice Guidelines*, 3rd ed. (Tampa, FL: International Research Foundation for RSD/CRPS, 2003), under "Importance of Objective Findings," www.rsdfoundation.org/en/en_clinical_practice_guidelines.html.

5.   Ibid.

6.   Tina A. Mohr, "Ho 'omaka ana e ola hou (Let the Healing Begin)," *Reflex Sympathetic Dystrophy Syndrome Association of America Newsletter*, 2003, 12–13, https://rsds.org/wp-content/uploads/2014/12/mohr.pdf.

7.   Ibid., 14.

8.   Ibid., 14–15.

9.   Derrick Phillips, "The Pain Returns," *Reflex Sympathetic Dystrophy Syndrome Association of America Newsletter*, 2010, n.p.

10.   Cleveland Clinic Foundation, "Reflex Sympathetic Dystrophy Syndrome," Cleveland Clinic, October 15, 2005, www.clevelandclinic.org/health/health-info/docs/2300/2307.asp?index=7577.

11.   Andrea Trescot, "Shingles and Interventional Pain Treatment," ASIPP News, 2006, 22–23, http://flsipp.org/FSIPPTrescotShingles.pdf.

12. Dorothee Sölle, *Suffering* (Minneapolis, MN: Fortress Press, 1989), 85.

13. "Multiple Sclerosis," Mayo Clinic, August 4, 2017, www.mayóclinic.org/diseases-conditions/multiple-sclerosis/symptoms-causes/syc-20350269.

14. Alessandro Clemenzi, Alessandra Pompa, Paolo Casillo, Luca Pace, Elio Troisi, Sheila Catani, and Maria Grazia Grasso, "Chronic Pain in Multiple Sclerosis: Is There Also Fibromyalgia? An Observational Study," *Medical Science Monitor* 20 (2014): 758–66, doi:10.12659/msm.890009. See also Saeed Talebzadeh Nick, Charles Roberts, Seth Billiodeaux, Debra Elliott Davis, Behrouz Zamanifekri, Mohammad Ali Sahraian, Nadejda Alekseeva, et al., "Multiple Sclerosis and Pain," *Neurological Research* 34, no. 9 (2012): 829–41, doi:10.1179/1743132812y.0000000082.

15. Clemenzi et al. "Chronic Pain in Multiple Sclerosis," 759.

16. Bishnu Subedi and George T. Grossberg, "Phantom Limb Pain: Mechanisms and Treatment Approaches," *Pain Research and Treatment* 2011 (2011): 1–8, doi:10.1155/2011/864605.

17. Mark W. Weatherall, "The Diagnosis and Treatment of Chronic Migraine," *Therapeutic Advances in Chronic Disease* 6, no. 3 (2015): 115–23, doi:10.1177/2040622315579627.

14. GETTING MOVING—EXERCISE AND PHYSICAL THERAPY

1. Academy of Medical Royal Colleges, *Exercise: The Miracle Cure and the Role of the Doctor in Promoting It* (London: Academy of Medical Royal Colleges, February 2015), www.aomrc.org.uk/wp-content/uploads/2016/05/Exercise_the_Miracle_Cure_0215.pdf.

2. U.K. Department of Health, *2009 Annual Report of the Chief Medical Officer.* (London: Department of Health, 2009), www.sthc.co.uk/Documents/CMO_Report_2009.pdf; H. Naci and J. P. A. Ioannidis, "Comparative Effectiveness of Exercise and Drug Interventions on Mortality Outcomes: Meta-epidemiological Study," *BMJ* 347 (2013), doi:10.1136/bmj.f5577; U. M. Kujala, "Evidence on the Effects of Exercise Therapy in the Treatment of Chronic Disease," *British Journal of Sports Medicine* 43, no. 8 (2009): 550–55, doi:10.1136/bjsm.2009.059808.

3. Silvano Mior, "Exercise in the Treatment of Chronic Pain," *Clinical Journal of Pain* 17, no. S4 (2002): 577, doi:10.1097/00002508-200112001-00016.

4. "More than 4 in 10 Cancers and Cancer Deaths Linked to Modifiable Risk Factors," American Cancer Society, www.cancer.org/latest-news/more-than-4-in-10-cancers-and-cancer-deaths-linked-to-modifiable-risk-factors.html.

5. Tormod Landmark, Pål Romundstad, Petter C. Borchgrevink, Stein Kaasa, and Ola Dale, "Associations between Recreational Exercise and Chronic Pain in the General Population: Evidence from the HUNT 3 Study," *Pain* 152, no. 10 (2011): 2241, doi:10.1016/j.pain.2011.04.029.

6. Vicki R. Harding, Maureen J. Simmonds, and Paul J. Watson, "Physical Therapy for Chronic Pain," *International Association for the Study of Pain* 6, no. 3 (1998): 1.

7. Ibid.

8. Ann E. Daly and Andrea Biolacerkowski, "Does Evidence Support Physiotherapy Management of Adult Complex Regional Pain Syndrome Type One? A Systematic Review," *European Journal of Pain* 13 (2009): 339, doi:10.1016/2008.05.003.

9. "Aquatic Exercises May Ease Fibromyalgia," *Washington Post* online, February 22, 2008, www.washingtonpost.com/wp-dyn/content/article/2008/02/22/AR2008022201922.html.

15. INTERVENTIONAL PAIN MANAGEMENT

1. T. T. Horlocker, D. J. Wedel, J. C. Rowlingson, F. K. Enneking, S. L. Kopp, H. T. Benzon, D. L. Brown, et al., "Regional Anesthesia in the Patient Receiving Antithrombotic or Thrombolytic Therapy: American Society of Regional Anesthesia and Pain Medicine Evidence-Based Guidelines (Third Edition)," *Regional Anesthesia and Pain Medicine* 35, no. 1 (January–February 2010): 64–101, www.ncbi.nlm.nih.gov/pubmed/20052816.

2. "Definition," North American Neuromodulation Society, www.neuromodulation.org/AboutNANS/Mission.aspx.

3. "Spinal Cord Stimulation," American Association of Neurological Surgeons, www.aans.org/Patients/Neurosurgical-Conditions-and-Treatments/Spinal-Cord-Stimulation.

4. Loz Blain, "Spinal Cord Stimulators—the 'Pacemaker' for Chronic Pain," *New Atlas*, August 12, 2009, http://newatlas.com/eon-mini-spinal-cord-stimulator/12486/.

5. Young Hoon Jeon, "Spinal Cord Stimulation in Pain Management: A Review," *Korean Journal of Pain* 25, no. 3 (2012): 143, doi:10.3344/kjp.2012.25.3.143.

6. Richard B. North, David H. Kidd, Farrokh Farrokhi, and Steven A. Piantadosi, "Spinal Cord Stimulation versus Repeated Lumbosacral Spine Surgery for Chronic Pain: A Randomized, Controlled Trial," *Neurosurgery* 56, no. 1 (2005): abstract, doi:10.1227/01.neu.0000144839.65524.e0.

7. Giancarlo Barolat, Beth Ketcik, and Jiping He, "Long-Term Outcome of Spinal Cord Stimulation for Chronic Pain Management," *Neuromodulation: Technology at the Neural Interface* 1, no. 1 (1998): abstract, doi:10.1111/j.1525-1403.1998.tb00027.x.

8. Konstantin Slavin, rev., "Peripheral Nerve Stimulation," International Neuromodulation Society, reviewed July 24, 2012, accessed April 4, 2017, www.neuromodulation.com/PNS.

9. P. D. Wall, "The Gate Control Theory of Pain Mechanisms: A Re-examination and Re-statement," *Pain* 6, no. 3 (1979): 388, doi:10.1016/0304-3959(79)90069-1; Laura Tyler Perryman, "Peripheral Nerve Stimulation and Percutaneous Electrical Nerve Stimulation in Pain Management: A Review and Update on Current Status," *International Journal of Pain & Relief*, December 18, 2017, www.scireslit.com/Pain/IJPR-ID17.pdf.

10. Mark D. Johnson and Kim J. Burchiel, "Peripheral Stimulation for Treatment of Trigeminal Postherpetic Neuralgia and Trigeminal Posttraumatic Neuropathic Pain: A Pilot Study," *Neurosurgery* 55, no. 1 (2004): 135–42, doi:10.1227/01.neu.0000126874.08468.89; Konstantin V. Slavin and Christian Wess, "Trigeminal Branch Stimulation for Intractable Neuropathic Pain: Technical Note," *Neuromodulation: Technology at the Neural Interface* 8, no. 1 (2005): 7–13, doi:10.1111/j.1094-7159.2005.05215.x; S. Amin, A. Buvanendran, K.-S. Park, Js. Kroin, and M. Moric, "Peripheral Nerve Stimulator for the Treatment of Supraorbital Neuralgia: A Retrospective Case Series," *Cephalalgia* 28, no. 4 (2008): 355–59, doi:10.1111/j.1468-2982.2008.01535.x; K. L. Reed, S. B. Black, C. J. Banta, and K. R. Will, "Combined Occipital and Supraorbital Neurostimulation for the Treatment of Chronic Migraine Headaches: Initial Experience," *Cephalalgia* 30, no. 3 (2009): 260–71, doi:10.1111/j.1468-2982.2009.01996.x; Brian Burns, "'Dual' Occipital and Supraorbital Nerve Stimulation for Primary Headache," *Cephalalgia* 30, no. 3 (2009): 257–59, doi:10.1111/j.1468-2982.2009.02000.x; Samer N. Narouze and Leonardo Kapural, "Supraorbital Nerve Electric Stimulation for the Treatment of Intractable Chronic Cluster Headache: A Case Report," *Headache: The Journal of Head and Face Pain* 47, no. 7 (2007): 1100–102, doi:10.1111/j.1526-4610.2007.00869.x; Lawrence W. Stinson, Grant T. Roderer, Nancy E. Cross, and Bennet E. Davis, "Peripheral Subcutaneous Electrostimulation for Control of Intractable Post-operative Inguinal Pain: A Case Report Series," *Neuromodulation: Technology at the Neural Interface* 4, no. 3 (2001): 99–104, doi:10.1046/j.1525-1403.2001.00099.x; Paul Verrills, Bruce Mitchell, David Vivian, and Chantelle Sinclair, "Peripheral Nerve Stimulation: A Treatment for Chronic Low Back Pain and Failed Back Surgery Syndrome?" *Neuromodulation: Technology at the Neural Interface* 12, no. 1 (2009): 68–75, doi:10.1111/j.1525-1403.2009.00191.x; Panagiotis Theodosiadis, Efthimios Samoladas, Vas-

ilios Grosomanidis, Teodor Goroszeniuk, and Sandesha Kothari, "A Case of Successful Treatment of Neuropathic Pain after a Scapular Fracture Using Subcutaneous Targeted Neuromodulation," *Neuromodulation: Technology at the Neural Interface* 11, no. 1 (2007): 62–65, doi:10.1111/j.1525-1403.2007.00144.x; Sandesha Kothari, "Neuromodulatory Approaches to Chronic Pelvic Pain and Coccygodynia," *Operative Neuromodulation: Acta Neurochirurgica Supplements* 97, pt. 1 (2007): 365–71, doi:10.1007/978-3-211-33079-1_48.

11.   Perryman, "Peripheral Nerve Stimulation."

12.   Ibid.

13.   El-Sayed A. Ghoname, William F. Craig, Paul F. White, Hesham E. Ahmed, Mohamed A. Hamza, Brent N. Henderson, Noor M. Gajraj, et al., "Percutaneous Electrical Nerve Stimulation for Low Back Pain," *JAMA* 281, no. 9 (1999): 818, doi:10.1001/jama.281.9.818.

14.   R. L. Weiner, C. M. Garcia, N. Vanquathem, "A Novel Miniature Wireless Neurostimulator in the Management of Chronic Craniofacial Pain: Preliminary Results from a Prospective Pilot Study," *Scandinavian Journal of Pain* 17 (October 2017): 350–54, doi:10.1016/j.sjpain.2017.09.010.

16. ALTERNATIVE MANAGEMENT OPTIONS

1.   Helen C. Ly, "Acupuncture and Chronic Pain," Psychology Department, Vanderbilt University, http://healthpsych.psy.vanderbilt.edu/HealthPsych/Acupuncture.htm.

2.   Anthea Levi, "How a Chiropractic Adjustment Led to Model Katie May's Death," Health.com, October 21, 2016, www.health.com/celebrities/chiropractic-adjustment-stroke-katie-may.

3.   "Man Suffers Stroke after Visit to Chiropractor," *Virginia Medical Law Report*, January 2018, https://valawyersweekly.com/vamedicallaw/.

4.   Brenda L. Griffith, "Massage Therapy and Pain Management," Practical Pain Management, last updated May 16, 2011, www.practicalpain management.com/treatments/manipulation/massage-therapy-pain-management.

5.   Suzanne Levy, "3 Ways Biofeedback Helps Patients Control Chronic Pain," *Health* online, last modified February 29, 2016, www.health.com/health/condition-article/0,,20189539,00.html.

6.   Rick Thomas, "EEG Biofeedback Training for Chronic Pain," RickThomasPHD.com, last modified 2008, www.rickdthomasphd.com/chronic_pain_treatment.

7. "Biofeedback: An Exciting and Personally Empowering Process," Life-Matters.com, accessed December 2009, www.lifematters.com/bfbarticle.html.

8. *Free Dictionary*, s.v. "cognitive-behavioral therapy," https://medical-dictionary.thefreedictionary.com/cognitive-behavioral therapy.

9. Dawn M. Ehde, Tiara M. Dillworth, and Judith A. Turner, "Cognitive-Behavioral Therapy for Individuals with Chronic Pain: Efficacy, Innovations, and Directions for Research," *American Psychologist* 69, no. 2 (February and March 2014): 161–62, doi:10.1037/a0035747.

17. MARIJUANA—THE MYSTERY DRUG

1. Z. Mehmedic, S. Chandra, D. Slade, et al., "Potency Trends of Δ9-THC and Other Cannabinoids in Confiscated Cannabis Preparations from 1993 to 2008," *Journal of Forensic Science* 55, no. 5 (2010): 1209–17.

2. W. C. Bunting, Lynda Garcia, and Ezekiel Edwards, *The War on Marijuana in Black and White* (New York: American Civil Liberties Union, June 2013), 123.

3. "Drug Facts: Marijuana," National Institute on Drug Abuse, February 2018, www.drugabuse.gov/publications/drugfacts/marijuana.

4. James Higdon, Jon Murray, Jack Shafer, Michael Grunwald, Mark Perry, Kevin Baker, Jaime Fuller, et al., "Jeff Sessions' Coming War on Legal Marijuana," *Politico*, December 5, 2016, www.politico.com/magazine/story/2016/12/jeff-sessions-coming-war-on-legal-marijuana-214501.

5. David Powell, Rosalie Liccardo Pacula, and Mireille Jacobson. "Do Medical Marijuana Laws Reduce Addiction and Deaths Related to Pain Killers?" Working Paper WR-1130, RAND Corporation, December 14, 2015, www.rand.org/pubs/working_papers/WR1130.html.

18. PAIN IN THE COURTROOM

1. Harold Merskey, "Pain Disorder, Hysteria or Somatization?" *Pain Research and Management* 9, no. 2 (2004): 67.

2. Michael Finch, "Law and the Problem of Pain," *University of Cincinnati Law Review* 74, no. 2 (2005): 284.

3. Johnny Cash, "Hurt," *American IV: The Man Comes Around* (American Recordings, 2002), MP3.

4. Frank T. Vertosick, *Why We Hurt: The Natural History of Pain* (New York: Harcourt, 2001), 224.

5.   Ananya Mandal, "History of Fibromyalgia," News Medical Life Sciences, last modified July 31, 2013, www.news-medical.net/health/History-of-Fibromyalgia.aspx.

6.   Eddie v. Unum Life Insurance Co., BCCA 507 (1999).

7.   Richard Hayles, "Defending Chronic Pain and Chronic Fatigue Claims," presented at "Managing and Litigating Disability Insurance Claims" (presentation at Managing and Litigating Disability and Insurance Claims Conference, Canadian Institute, Toronto, ON, October 21 and 22, 2010).

8.   Ibid.

9.   Michael Finch, "Law and the Problem of Pain," *University of Cincinnati Law Review* 74, no. 2 (2005).

10.   Ibid.

11.   Kenneth Mitchell, "The Dance of the Invisible Impairments: Chronic Pain Syndrome and the Disability Insurer," *American Society of Chronic Pain Newsletter*, October 2000, 1, www.workrxgroup.com/Research/The%20Dance%20of%20the%20Invisible%20Impairments.pdf.

12.   "Chronic Pain and Social Security Disability Insurance," TrueHelp, www.truehelp.com/understanding-ssdi/guidelines-by-disability/chronic-pain-and-social-security-disability/.

13.   Tim Moore, Social Security Disability Resource Center, www.ssdrc.com/.

14.   Dennis Thompson, "Will Insurance Cover Your Pain Treatment?" Everyday Health, last modified March 9, 2010, www.everydayhealth.com/pain-management/will-insurance-cover-your-chronic-pain-treatment.aspx.

15.   Ibid.

16.   Ibid.

19. COEXISTING WITH PAIN

1.   Frank T. Vertosick Jr., *Why We Hurt: The Natural History of Pain* (San Diego, CA: Harvest Books, 2001), 229

2.   Charles Swanson, ed., *Mayo Clinic on Chronic Pain* (Phoenix, AZ: Mayo Clinic, 2002).

3.   Vertosick, *Why We Hurt*.

4.   Chris Wells, Graham Nown, and Ronald Melzack, *The Pain Relief Handbook: Self-Health Methods for Managing Pain* (Toronto: Firefly Books, 1998).

5.   Ibid.

6.   Kelly McGonigal, "Yoga for Chronic Pain," IdeaFit.com, last modified June 1, 2006, www.ideafit.com/fitness-library/yoga-for-chronic-pain.

7. Swanson, *Mayo Clinic on Chronic Pain*, 29.

8. Susan L. Gardner, "Introduction to the 12 Step Program for Chronic Pain," *ZebraMichelle* (blog), August 21, 2012, https://zebrami-chelle.wordpress.com/category/12-steps-for-chronic-pain/.

20. TOWARD A PAIN-FREE FUTURE

1. Patricia H. Berry and June L. Dahl, "The New JCAHO Pain Standards: Implications for Pain Management Nurses," *Pain Management Nursing* 1, no. 1 (2000): 3–4, doi:10.1053/jpmn.2000.5833.

2. Joint Commission, "Facts about the Joint Commission," Joint Commission website, www.jointcommission.org/facts_about_the_joint_commission/.

3. Ibid.

4. Michael W. Smith, "Chronic Pain: New Research, New Treatments," WebMD, www.webmd.com/pain-management/features/chronic-pain-new-research-new-treatments#1.

5. National Center for Complementary and Integrative Health, "NIH Analysis Shows Americans Are in Pain," National Center for Complementary and Integrative Health, National Institutes of Health, August 11, 2015, https://nccih.nih.gov/news/press/08112015.

6. Michael W. Smith, "Chronic Pain: New Research, New Treatments," WebMD, www.webmd.com/pain-management/features/chronic-pain-new-research-new-treatments#1.

7. David Kannerstein, "Changing Thoughts and Beliefs about Pain," http://drdavidkannerstein.com/changing.html (site discontinued).

8. Linda Brown, interview by ABC Nightly News (October 2011).

9. Ibid.

10. Robert M. Califf, "21st Century Cures Act: Making Progress on Shared Goals for Patients," *FDA Voice*, U.S. Food and Drug Administration, December 13, 2016, https://blogs.fda.gov/fdavoice/index.php/2016/12/21st-century-cures-act-making-progress-on-shared-goals-for-patients/.

11. "Pfizer and Lilly Receive FDA Fast Track Designation for Tanezumab," Pfizer, June 13, 2017, www.pfizer.com/news/press-release/press-release-detail/pfizer_and_lilly_receive_fda_fast_track_designation_for_tanezumab.

12. Andres Jara-Oseguera, Sidney A. Simon, and Tamara Rosenbaum, "TRPV1: On the Road to Pain Relief," *Current Molecular Pharmacology* 1, no. 3 (2008), abstract, www.eurekaselect.com/openurl/content.php?genre=article&issn=1874-4672&volume=1&issue=3&spage=255.

13. Burel Goodin, Timothy Ness, and Meredith Robbins, "Oxytocin—a Multifunctional Analgesic for Chronic Deep Tissue Pain," *Current Pharma-*

ceutical Design 21, no. 7 (2014): 906–13, doi:10.2174/1381612820666
141027111843.

14.   Amy R. Tso and Peter J. Goadsby, "Anti-CGRP Monoclonal Antibodies: The Next Era of Migraine Prevention?" *Current Treatment Options in Neurology* 19, no. 8 (2017): abstract. See also Peter J. Goadsby, Lars Edvinsson, and R. Ekman, "Vasoactive Peptide Release in the Extracerebral Circulation of Humans during Migraine Headache," *Annals of Neurology* 28, no. 2 (1990): 183–87, doi:10.1002/ana.410280213; Peter J. Goadsby and Lars Edvinsson, "The Trigeminovascular System and Migraine: Studies Characterizing Cerebrovascular and Neuropeptide Changes Seen in Humans and Cats," *Annals of Neurology* 33, no. 1 (1993): 48–56, doi:10.1002/ana.410330109; G. Juhasz, T. Zsombok, B. Jakab, J. Nemeth, J. Szolcsanyi, and G. Bagdy, "Sumatriptan Causes Parallel Decrease in Plasma Calcitonin Gene-Related Peptide (CGRP) Concentration and Migraine Headache during Nitroglycerin Induced Migraine Attack," *Cephalalgia* 25, no. 3 (2005): 179–83, doi:10.1111/j.1468-2982.2005.00836.x.

15.   Peter J. Goadsby, Uwe Reuter, Yngve Hallström, Gregor Broessner, Jo H. Bonner, Feng Zhang, Sandhya Sapra, Hernan Picard, Daniel D. Mikol, and Robert A. Lenz, "A Controlled Trial of Erenumab for Episodic Migraine," *New England Journal of Medicine* 377, no. 22 (2017): abstract, doi:10.1056/nejmoa1705848.

16.   Ibid.

INDEX

Abdul, Paula, 62
ablation procedures, 126
Academy of Medical Royal Colleges
    (AOMRC), 115–116
acetaminophen, 10; FDA on death from,
    11; side effects of, 11
acupuncture, 135
acute pain: as alert system, 41; chronic
    pain compared to, 36, 43, 46, 63, 118;
    opioids for, 25
Adams, Henry, 82
addiction, 30–31; anecdote on, 15–16;
    defined by ASAM, 29–30; dependence
    compared to, 17–18; history as red
    flag, 19; OBOT for opioid, 31–32; to
    opioids, 12–13, 16–17;
    pseudoaddiction, 18–19; relapse with,
    32
addiction treatment: incarceration
    compared to cost of, 33; medication
    for, 29–30, 30; National Institute on
    Drug Abuse and NIH on, 32, 33;
    OBOT for, 31–32
ADiseaseADay.com, 97
African Americans, 52–53
alcohol: with drugs, 24; self-medicating
    with, 69
allodynia: CSS and, 99; RSD/CRPS and,
    105
alternative therapy, 122, 123; acupuncture
    as, 135; biofeedback as, 133–134,

138–139, 140; CBT as, 133–134, 138,
    139–140; chiropractics as, 136; for
    chronic pain, 133–134; Internet and,
    134; massage as, 137–138; skepticism
    for, 134; surgery compared to, 151
American Society of Addiction Medicine
    (ASAM): addiction defined by, 29–30;
    on overdose, 30–31
anecdotes: on addiction, 15–16; on
    expectations, 83; on fibromyalgia
    diagnosis, 95–96, 153–154; on
    language barrier, 49; on obesity, 73; on
    physical therapy, 119–120; on RSD/
    CRPS management, 104
anesthesiology, 6–7
anesthetic, local, 125–126
antidepressants, 69
AOMRC. *See* Academy of Medical Royal
    Colleges
aquatic exercise, 122–123
Aristotle, 113
ASAM. *See* American Society of
    Addiction Medicine

"Bankruptcies of the Heart: Secondary
    Losses from Disabling Chronic Pain"
    (Bedard), 59–60
BCBS. *See* Blue Cross Blue Shield
Bedard, Marcia, 59–60; on secondary gain
    theory, 60, 62; on sympathy, 60–61
Beecher, Henry Ward, 41

ABOUT THE AUTHOR

Akhtar Purvez, MD, is a physician and researcher who works and lives in Virginia. He was clinical adjunct professor at Lincoln Memorial University, Tennessee, and has been involved in training physician assistants, medical students, residents, fellows, and other physicians in pain management and addiction-related issues. He supports pain advocacy, pain policy, training, and research. Dr. Purvez writes and speaks on these issues on radio and television, including on local ABC and NBC stations. He has numerous scientific papers to his credit, in addition to a chapter on pain management in *The American College of Physicians (ACP) Manual of Critical Care*.